PUBLIC HEALTH PROFITEERING

PUBLIC HEALTH PROFITEERING

James T. Bennett
Thomas J. DiLorenzo

Transaction Publishers
New Brunswick (U.S.A.) and London (U.K.)

This book is printed on acid-free paper that meets the American National Standard for Permanence of Paper for Printed Library Materials.

Library of Congress Catalog Number: 2001027886
ISBN: 0–7658–0074–8
Printed in the United States of America

Library of Congress Cataloging-in-Publication Data

Bennett, James T.
Public health profiteering / James T. Bennett and Thomas J. DiLorenzo.
p. cm.
Includes bibliographical references and index.
ISBN 0-7658-0074-8 (alk. paper)
1. Koop, C. Everett (Charles Everett), 1916—Biography. 2. Health officers—United States—Biography. 3. Pediatric surgeons—United States—Biography. I. DiLorenzo, Thomas J. II. Title.

RA5.K66 B46 2001
610'.92—dc21
[B]

2001027886

Contents

Acknowledgment

The diet industry which feeds on the hopes and the fears of those who need—or think that they need—to lose weight has been growing fat for more than a century. According to a story in the "Style" section of the *Washington Post* on October 12, 1999, the first known diet book, *Letter on Corpulence*, was published in 1864 by William Banting, a casketmaker who had become so fat that he could no longer tie his shoes. His prescription for obesity: booze and foods low in carbohydrates. Nearly 60,000 copies were sold, and diets of one sort or another have been touted ever since. The record shows that many of those who have condemned obesity were themselves overweight to a greater or lesser degree. Those Who Know Better never hesitate to tell the great unwashed to "do as I say, not as I do."

This book is about C. Everett Koop, the idol of Those Who Know Best in the field of public health. Arguably, no one has preached to the great unwashed with greater hypocrisy and sanctimony. As examples, Koop reviles obesity, but is overweight by his own admission; he vilifies demon alcohol, but drinks multiple martinis; and he condemns tobacco in every form, yet smoked a pipe for years after the Surgeon General's report on tobacco. Koop rails against commercialism in medicine and virtually every other form, but never seems to pass up a chance to sell (or rent) his own reputation. He has shilled, lobbied, hawked, and endorsed products for a host of firms: Wyeth Ayerst (the people who brought us fen-phen), Weight Watchers, Jenny Craig, Glaxo-Wellcome, BioPure, Neurocrine, Time Life, Kelloggs, First Circle Medical, Intel, WRP Corporation, and the list goes on on. . . . He Knows What Is Good for Us and has pocketed a king's ransom from his high-handed hectoring.

We thank the Sunmark Foundation for generous research support that made this book possible and the Locke Institute; excellent research assistance was provided by Mattias Eng, Christoper Farris, and Meghan O'Brien. We are especially grateful to Bill Kauffman whose editorial skills and wonderful sense of the absurd contributed so much to this work. Of course, we alone are responsible for any errors.

Finally, one point must be made explicit: No individual company, industry group, or commercial interest of any sort contributed financially or in any other way to the research, writing, publishing, sales, or distribution of this book. We have no links whatsoever to tobacco, snack foods, fast-food companies, distillers, vintners, brewers, or any other politically incorrect (or, for that matter, politically correct) economic, social, or political interest.

1

The Very Model of a Modern Surgeon General: How a Brilliant Pediatric Surgeon Became an Annoying and Sanctimonious Nanny

"Physician, heal thyself."

—Luke, IV, 23

"I am the very model of a modern [surgeon] general, I've information vegetable, animal, and mineral . . . "

—W.S. Gilbert, *The Pirates of Penzance*

It always comes back to the uniform. That absurd, gold-braided, three-starred, ill-fitting vice admiral's outfit. "I admit that unlike some of my predecessors, I enjoyed wearing my uniform,"[1] he confessed. The wearer must have believed that he derived magical powers from this livery; the coat, or so he thought, conferred unimpeachable dignity upon him whom it cloaked. He had never served in the real military, and that gap in his record seemed to gnaw at him. So he wore the comic-opera costume of the Surgeon General, striding down the corridors of influence like a Patton, a MacArthur, a Rommel. Mere human rules and codes of conduct no longer applied to him: he became brusque, imperious, peremptory, and would eventually demand that when he departs this vale of tears, his body be interred in Arlington National Cemetery—an honor for which his silly uniform did not qualify him. He cracked his knuckles when meeting with others, an act of rudeness, to be sure, but he was no simple doctor saving one life at a time—he was SURGEON GENERAL. He didn't have time to be polite! He would save us all, by golly, and if the occasional recalcitrant smoker or fugitive fatty objected, well, you can't make an omelete without breaking a few eggs.

The longer he wore the uniform, the more convinced he became that he was, in fact, a general, leading his army of public health administrators against the formidable enemy . . . only the enemy was protean, it wore many faces: sometimes it took the familiar malevolent form of a virus, a disease, but at other times it assumed the disquieting countenance of the American people. Yes, the American people. The longer he wore the stars and gold braids, the more he realized: the people were stupid, feckless, improvident, unable to make the simplest decisions about their lives. They were lousy parents, too, and so the Surgeon General had no choice but to take the battle to the schools, for as he said in a moment of Olympian candor, "Like Communists, you have to get them when they're young."[2]

Slowly, but surely, the Surgeon General began to speak in the language of war. We could write this off as metaphorical excess, as when an overly ardent football coach speaks of his team as if they are about to refight Gettysburg, but the difference is this: the football coach is guiding a couple of dozen volunteers in an hour-long game; the Surgeon General—if he is able to make effective use of his bully pulpit, and no one ever put the bully into bully pulpit like our subject—has at his disposal the police power of the U.S. government. Disobey the laws or federal regulations that he is able to convince Congress to pass or the President to issue, and you'll wind up wearing a uniform of your own. It has no gold braids or pretty stars, but it does have a number stitched into the shirt.

To the rest of us, at least at first, the Surgeon General was an object of mirth. The beard, reminiscent of an old Dutch patriarch, was a somewhat endearing archaism, like a handlebar mustache or periwig. As for the uniform, who could gaze upon it without cracking a smile? He was called an "admiral in the Ruritanian navy." Strangers at airports asked him, "Skycap, can you take my bag, please?" and "Is Flight 726 to Omaha on time?"[3] He bore these unintended insults with equanimity. Most of us are equipped with inner detectors that go clang-a-lang when we are making an ass of ourselves; the Surgeon General's ass detector was broken, or perhaps he taught himself to ignore it. A righteous man, after all, is bound to be misunderstood by his benighted neighbors.

And C. Everett Koop, the fourteenth Surgeon General of the United States, is nothing if not righteous. But he is more: a righteous hypocrite, for starters. It was often said—by himself, especially—that Koop left office in possession of the one commodity that cannot be manufactured in Washington: integrity. He bathed in honor, he was lathered with ennoblement, he reeked of integrity. Or so the story went. Upon leaving office, he declared himself to be "the health conscience of America."[4] He was America's family doctor, the Marcus Welby of these United States, and other silly sobriquets, often minted by the ever-active Koop publicity machine. (Have you ever heard an actual American refer to Koop as her "family doctor"?) He spared no opportunity to announce that he would not, no not ever in a million years, cash in on his Washington experience. Which of course is the precise strategy that one follows if one wishes to cash in on one's Washington experience, but good.

"As I came to the end of my Surgeon General years, I felt that I had gained the public's trust and that I should do something with it. First, I wanted to make sure I did not use that trust only for private gain."[5] Note the Clintonesque qualifier "only." It is significant, for like most New Year's resolutions, this soon passed into nothingness, and Koop was raking in the dough hand over fist. For C. Everett Koop has since cashed in on whatever trust he had won from the American people. He has been a shill for killer diet drugs. He has hyped the unhealthy thinness craze—to his own profit. He has been subsidized by pharmaceutical companies. His foundation has fattened itself at the public trough, as the Clinton-Gore administration funneled money to a Koop organization to do work that others were already doing—without public alms. Having gotten what he could from the Republicans, who rammed through his controversial 1981 nomination as Surgeon General, he has since played footsies with the Democrats, finding soulmates (and patrons) in Hillary Rodham Clinton and Vice President Albert Gore, Jr. ("I always do everything Dr. Koop tells me,"[6] cooed the First Lady as she helped her fitness guru launch yet another lucrative scam, with the imperative Hillary-esque title "Shape Up, America!") Integrity, Dr. Koop has found, can be very useful collateral in the world of politics. Especially when the media love you, and alchemize anything you leave in your wake into chicken salad and lemonade.

* * *

Charles Everett Koop was the son of a prosperous banker in the Flatbush section of Brooklyn. He was an only child, a bit of a weirdo, by all accounts, who was picked on by his classmates. From his earliest days he wanted to be a doctor. As a teenager, he picked up stray cats, anesthetized them, and removed their ovaries—all in good clean fun, he assures us, despite the apparent ghoulishess.[7] (Seventy years later, he would do public-service announcements praising the use of animals in medical research. In this, at least, Koop has exhibited an unwavering consistency.)

He seems to have had an uncanny knack for drawing precisely the wrong lesson from the experiences of his boyhood. For instance, during Prohibition he reports being "caught in the crossfire of gang warfare on Fourteenth Street right in front of my house."[8] One gang member was killed. Thankfully, young Koop was unharmed, and he would grow into an influential adult who recommended a variety of neo-Prohibitionist measures to combat whichever habits and vices he disliked. Including, incredibly, alcohol, despite the taste he would develop for hard liquor.

The lad could endure only so many beatings from the neighborhood toughs, and his mother eventually enrolled him in the tony private Flatbush School. From there it was off to Dartmouth, where he picked up a nickname. Now, the boy had always hated the name Everett, so one might think he would welcome a manly moniker like "Butch" or "Ace" or "Duke." Alas, the Dartmouth wits dubbed him "Chick"—get it?; as in "Chick[en]" Koop—and he tried mightily, but without success, to shed this infra dig nickname. For it stuck. (Don't try calling him "Chick" today or you'll get the same searing stare that the formidable second Mrs. Dole fixes on those clods who call her "Liddy.")

At this time his father performed an admirable act from which young C.E.—heaven forfend that we call him Everett or Chick—extracted the wrong lesson. As Koop tells it in his autobiography, grandly titled *Koop: The Memoirs of America's Family Doctor*:

> Once, when I was home from college for a weekend, my mother approached me in the pantry:
>
> "What are we going to do about your father's smoking? He smokes almost three packs a day, coughs all the time, and I'm certain he's shortening his life."
>
> I replied, "Forget it, Mom. Pop hasn't got the guts to stop smoking."
>
> That was a stupid, sophomoric thing for me to say, because I was talking about a man who had once pulled out his own decayed teeth with pliers, without anesthetic. As I thoughtlessly dismissed Dad's ability to stop smoking, he quietly

> stepped into the room without my knowing it and overheard what I said. Without a word, he turned around, went upstairs, threw his cigarettes in the toilet, and wrapped up all of his smoking paraphernalia, never to smoke again in his life.[9]

A striking story, and a real testament to his father. Yet the son seems not to have derived the correct lesson from Pop's act of will-power. No coercion, no sin taxes, no prohibition of the demon weed was necessary to get Pop to go cold turkey. Rather, moral and family suasion did the trick; a bit of shame, a macho dare, and Pop simply quit. But just as the disrespectful son doubted that his father had the "guts" to stop smoking, so too does he disbelieve in the capacity of his fellow citizens to refrain from potentially injurious behavior on their own. They need a push, a pull, a prod from Uncle Sam—and the stern visage of Dr. Koop, prod in hand, hovering above us. "[T]he public has to become educated,"[10] is a typical Koopian declaration, and he leaves no doubt about who is to be the educator and who is to be the educatee.

He was a fanatical anti-smoker from the beginning, viewing a few puffs on the nicotine stick as evidence of the deepest moral failing. He was a moralist and a bully, even when other boys were calling him Chick. Most men, when recalling when first they laid eyes on the woman to whom they would plight their troth, remember a word, a glance, a gesture, a whiff of perfume, the sight of their future wife walking down a lane with the breeze teasing her hair. Not our Chick. His tender memory goes like this: "Like many college women in the thirties, Betty was toying with the idea of taking up smoking. In the course of our first conversation I happened to say that I would never be interested in any girl who smoked. After hearing that, she never took a puff."[11]

First Pa, then Betty. By insult or threat, young Mr. Koop had deterred two intimates from this nasty habit. If the children of the baby boom learned anything from thousands of hours spent watching family sitcoms on the idiot box, it was never to give in to a bully: he feeds on acquiescence. Resist and he'll back down. Alas, the failure of Pa Koop and the lovely Betty only emboldened Chick, and set him upon a lifetime of officious meddling.

Boys who experiment on feline cadavers likely end up in one of two professions: surgery or serial killing. Koop chose the former, thankfully, and was graduated from Cornell University Medical College. Columbia rejected him, a slight that seems to have rankled for half a century. He uses it as the prop in the sort of self-congratulatory humor masquerading as self-deprecation that is the currency of the insecure. "Recently, while making some TV shows at Columbia," he said in his post-SG period, "I told the president of the medical center that if Columbia had admitted me in 1937, I might have made something of myself. He agreed."[12] Heh-heh-heh. There is something pathetic about an eighty-year-old man, nationally prominent, a leader in his fields of endeavor, feeling the need to pat himself on the back. Especially given the fawning, nay, suctorial, press that he has received for over a dozen years. He might just as well have praised himself for his ability to convert his reputation into a ready and steady flow of cash—but the good doctor is rather less willing to joke about his facility at *that* skill.

The newly minted Dr. Koop did his internship at the University of Pennsylvania Hospital in Philadelphia. A war was on, and while other doctors entered military service Chick stayed behind to fight "the Battle of Spruce Street,"[13] as they joked. There was nothing ignoble about this—doctors were needed just as much on the home front as they were in the European or Pacific theaters of operation—but his failure to join the armed forces was something of a botheration to Koop. It may well explain the severe case of khaki-envy that he later manifested in his wearing of the Surgeon General's uniform and his bizarre request to be buried in Arlington National Cemetery, amidst the acres and acres of men who wore other than the uniforms of a comic opera.

Let us be clear and fair: by all accounts, C. Everett Koop was an outstanding surgeon. Only a stone could read stories of his work with children in his pre-political career without welling eyes. He answered his calling, and he honored it. After his internship was completed, Koop became surgeon-in-chief of the Children's Hospital in Philadelphia. Pediatric surgery was a new field; Koop was a pioneer, a brash, intelligent pathbreaker. The lack of respect accorded pediatric surgery nettled him; forty-five years later, he still complained about the dingy office he had been assigned. He invented any number of surgical techniques, and as he later wrote, immodestly but accurately, "As a physician, I have always been at least a crusader, at best a pioneer."[14] If only he had remained a physician.

C. Everett Koop became an evangelical Christian during these years. He was a particularly eloquent leader of the right-to-life movement; his views were informed by his work with severely handicapped infants and children, and no matter how one comes down on the morality and legality of abortion, Koop's labors on behalf of these most vulnerable of children demands respect. As he asked, "How could I ever accept the destruction of the unborn after a career devoted to the repair of imperfect newborns, knowing the joy and fulfillment they brought to their families?"[15]

Koop was raising a family himself in these years, though "raising" may be overstating the case. He and the smoke-free Betty had four children. Now, even in the best of circumstances a surgeon's time with his family is going to be limited, but Dr. Koop's crusading zeal made him scarcer than most physician-fathers. He spent Sundays supervising the provision of medical aid to indigent Philadelphians; this task consumed Sundays from noon to midnight. He was an absentee father, albeit one who was performing good works. "My mistake was that I did not spend as much time with my family as I did with the homeless,"[16] he later regretted, but it could not have been otherwise. A zealot always seems to prefer the presence of strangers in need of ministration to intimacy. He may try to save the world but perhaps let his backyard go to seed. Such zeal may be quite useful down any number of avenues—but not in service to the state, and that, alas, is where this Chick eventually came to roost.

"After thirty-five years at Children's Hospital espousing the cause of the disenfranchised and fighting for a fairer deal for children, I wanted to enter a larger arena and fight on behalf of a broader constituency,"[17] is how Koop explains his plunge into politics. This explanation is riddled with the usual cant, and it diminishes the very real good that Koop the private citizen had done. He saved lives, for goodness sake, and made it possible for little ones born with what once were disabling deformities to live better lives. What line of work could possibly be nobler? But to Koop the politico, his doctoring now seems like mere "espousing" and "fighting" for a "constituency." These are the phrases of politics, used by special pleaders, Beltway bandits, and lobbyists. He was not "fighting" for his patients, he was healing them. But such is the way of Potomac fever: he who contracts this usually incurable ailment comes to perhaps view his erstwhile activities in private life as unimportant and trivial, the merest crumb when compared to the higher calling of securing funding, offering bought-and-paid-for testimony, and hobnobbing with people who know Ted Koppel.

Koop had already been infected with the celebrity virus, albeit in a fairly benign form. He and the theologian Francis Schaeffer had made a series of films called *Whatever Happened to the Human Race*? These were powerful, if unsubtle, attacks on abortion and euthanasia. They even produced a memorable tableau: Koop, wearing his best Old Testament scowl, standing on an island in the Dead Sea, surrounded by thousands of bobbing dolls representing the victims of abortion. This was also Sodom and Gomorrah territory, though in later years Koop would downplay his evangelical Christian aversion to the acts that led God to vaporize those ancient dens of iniquity.

The handful of liberals who saw *Whatever Happened to the Human Race*? gaped in horror, but at this stage in his pre-political career, Koop wouldn't give a pillar of salt for their good opinion. The five films Koop made with Schaeffer turned him into a star on the Christian Right, a veritable Charlton Heston or Dean Jones. He came to the attention of the New Right, which was surging just as Koop was getting used to the idea of himself as sagacious celebrity.

The transformation of Chick Koop from benevolent healer to wheeler-dealer began ominously enough, with an August 1980 phone call from an aide to Senator Jesse Helms. "Don't you think it's time the Surgeon General was a surgeon?" asked the factotum. Koop, sixty-four, preparing to retire from the University of Pennsylvania School of Medicine, was speechless—for perhaps the last time in his life. For "like most Americans, I didn't think about the Surgeon General very much, if at all."[18] If only this were still so. If only Dr. Koop had kept on not thinking very much about it. But once in office, after a nasty confirmation fight in which his pro-life position won him vilification from folks like Sen. Ted Kennedy (D-MA), who soon would be hailing him as the best thing to happen to medicine since we learned that penicillin cured the clap, Koop treated this brummagem job as a cross between Pope, Secretary of State, and Exalted Ruler of the Universe.

The day after Ronald Reagan defeated Jimmy Carter for the presidency, Dr. Koop called the Helms operative—with whom he had previously been a bit coy—and declared that he was "enthusiastically seeking"[19] the job of Surgeon General. Thus began an almost year-long battle between Koop and the forces of enlightened liberalism: Congressman Henry Waxman (D-CA), Senator Kennedy (D-MA), the *New York Times*, and others Who Know Best. The *Times* sneered that he was "Dr. Unqualified," an "affront to the public health profession and to the public."[20] (Technically, Dr. Koop *was* unqualified for the post. By law, a Surgeon General could be no older than sixty-four years and twenty-nine days: when nominated, Koop was several months older. The age limit was removed after some legislative wrangling, though one lowlight was the sixty-eight-year-old Speaker of the House, Thomas P. ["Tip"] O'Neill [D-MA], defending what appeared to be rank age discrimination.)

Planned Parenthood, the National Abortion Rights Action League, and the lovely ladies of the National Organization for Women demanded that the Senate reject Dr. Koop. Many of these nemeses would later change their minds, when finally they figured out that Koop was no right-wing bogeyman but rather an inveterate, puritanical busybody, a bluenose and snoop who could know no rest as long as a single American was eating, drinking, or smoking a substance of which he disapproved. (Of Cong. Waxman, the most reflexively knee-jerk advocate of federal regulation of every aspect of human health, a man who said "Koop scares me," the forgiving doctor would later gush that he "was good for the country."[21])

You might ask, "Why do we even *need* a Surgeon General of the United States?" An outstanding question, though the mere asking of it disqualifies you from occupying any position within the boundaries of the District of Columbia.

In 1870, Treasury Secretary George S. Boutwell of the ethically challenged administration of President U.S. Grant proposed, and the Congress assented, to create a "Supervising Surgeon of the Marine Hospital Service" to oversee medical care for ancient mariners and other deserving seamen. There is no evidence that John M. Woodworth, the first Supervising Surgeon General (the military suffix was added in 1873) worried overly much about second-hand smoke; he was busy enough reforming the patronage-ridden system of marine hospitals along civil-service lines. Venereal disease was a fairly constant concern of the early Surgeon Generals, sailors on leave so often exhibiting the morals of tomcats and Kennedys, but for the most part the Surgeon General and the Public Health Service that he led aimed their fire at yellow fever, leprosy, and influenza. Of course there were the usual spurts of expansion and efforts to redefine "public health" in a way that brought more and more private citizens under the watchful eye of government doctors: the Public Health Service took to funding state and local health departments (and thus bringing far-flung medical communities under Washington's thumb) and became "doctor to the Indians of America"[22] in 1955. The PHS was placed within the Federal Security Agency in 1939; the FSA eventually mutated into the Department of Health and Human Services we all love today.

The high-water mark of the position, pre-Koop, had been the 1964 report on the hazards of smoking by Surgeon General Luther Terry, who declared at a press conference, "Cigarette smoking is causally related to lung cancer in men," thus beginning a now almost four-decades long crusade by the federal government against the cancer stick—a crusade that began with the provision of information and seems likely to end in prohibition. Terry's news conference, by the way, was held on a Saturday, "to minimize the impact on tobacco stocks."[23] (Koop went to bat to get Terry, who died in 1985, buried with full honors in Arlington National Cemetery. "He certainly affected—and saved—more lives than many of the generals buried there,"[24] said Koop, who later tried—unsuccessfully—to pull strings to secure for himself the same honor.)

The Surgeon General's bailiwick has grown to include about 5,500 active-duty officers who range from dentists to veterinarians; these officers people agencies including the Centers for Disease Control, the Food and Drug Administration, Indian Health Service, National Institutes of Health, and the Alcohol, Drug Abuse, and Mental Health Administration, among others. As for purview, after C. Everett Koop, the sky appears to be the limit: gun control, movies, marijuana, hamburgers: there is nothing the Surgeon General can't examine and propose to ban—or at least heavily tax.

Fortunately for American liberties, the post-Koop Surgeon Generals and nominees have been less adept than Koop at winning fawning media coverage. President Clinton's first Surgeon General, Jocelyn Elders, was among the more colorful of the Arkansas Travelers he brought to Washington. In an administration given to weasel words and circumlocution Elders possessed the rare virtue of frankness, but her seeming to place the imprimatur of the U.S. government on teenage masturbation struck many Americans as a mite too frank. (The kids seem to learn this skill fairly well without Uncle Sam's helping hand.) Elders's would-be successor, Dr. Henry Foster, had performed numerous abortions on as well as sterilizations of poor women, and so seemed less like America's doctor than perhaps a doctor imported from Aldous Huxley's *Brave New World*. Foster foundered, and Clinton finally came up with a candidate who could survive the Senate, Dr. David Satcher, former president of Meharry Medical College in Nashville, who won confirmation despite his opposition to a ban on the controversial procedure known as a partial-birth abortion.

All this partisan wrangling inspired Dr. Koop, no longer a callow naif gone to Washington but a certified Wise Man, to suggest to President Clinton that "There should be a law that says this person [the Surgeon General] would be apolitical and when he is appointed, he will not be answerable to the President for what he says about health or anything else."[25] This is a classic Wise Man prescription: remove politics from government, and turn government over to the Best and Brightest—or should we say Best-Connected and Brightest by the standards that make ciphers like Clark Clifford and Vernon Jordan into virtual Solomons. But we are getting ahead of ourselves. For no one ever politicized the position of Surgeon General like that apostle of the apolitical, C. Everett Koop.

"[B]y 1980 the Surgeon General's position had become essentially moribund," notes Koop. "It had been left vacant under the Nixon presidency, and under Carter it had been combined with the job of assistant secretary of health in the Department of Health and Human Services."[26] This speaks well of the Nixon and Carter administrations—perhaps those much-maligned men were capable of acting wisely on occasion—but the fearsome budget-cutters of the Reagan administration had high hopes for a reinvigorated Surgeon General. He was to spearhead the nation's moral revival and place a medical stamp of approval on the agenda of the pro-family and pro-life movements. At least that's what the Reaganites told their supporters in those communities. A somewhat more cynical view is that they needed to throw a sop to their ardent but politically unsophisticated troops, and what could be soppier than appointing a strange-looking and seemingly apolitical doctor to the insignificant post of Surgeon General? The pro-lifers are propitiated, and the merely symbolic nature of the appointment does not detract from the broader economic and foreign policy objectives of the administration.

Koop had other ideas. He was neither sop nor sap; he imagined himself as a beribboned general in the vanguard of "medical leadership, especially in the education of the public about the promotion of health and the prevention of disease."[27] The "role of federal medicine," he declared, is "to lead, not merely to follow."[28] This would come as news to Koop's fellow pioneers in medical research: the great breakthroughs of our day—Jonas Salk's polio vaccine, Michael De Bakey's artificial heart—have been made by doctors who were private citizens, not GS-something federal employees serving time for Uncle Sam and wearing funny uniforms.

The contentious debate over his appointment was ended; the doctor was in. He now held the rank of vice admiral, and for the first time since he was a Boy Scout he donned a uniform. His Potomac fever raged; the only cure, voluntary exile from the seat of power, was out of the question. "Now I realized that my life would change at least once an hour throughout each coming day, perhaps as often as fifteen minutes," he exulted. The saving of children, the repair and reconstruction of the injured and ill, began to seem like small potatoes. Koop was intoxicated by the thrill of being at the center of the known universe. "With a sense of excitement and humility [*sic*—oh my! is this ever a *sic*!], I realized that each day I was doing something that was counting not just for me, not just for now, but for the entire country, and for maybe an endless time ahead."[29] This gives hubris a bad name: the pediatric surgeon had become a wee bit power-mad. "Endless time ahead"? And things would only get worse.

"As Surgeon General, I took as my mission nothing less than improving the health of the entire nation,"[30] declared Dr. Koop, who had obviously lost his humility somewhere north of I-495. His predecessors he regarded largely as ciphers, as well-meaning but ultimately ineffectual doctors who failed to compass the majesty of their vice admiralty. Except for Luther Terry.

Terry got good press for his 1964 report on smoking; Koop, who had been battered by the media during his confirmation battle, decided to bolster his reputation by following in Terry's footsteps—sort of. For whereas Luther Terry relied on incontrovertible evidence that long-term cigarette smoking *can* be harmful to one's health, our man Koop, the "entire country" his patient, his vision stretching for "an endless time ahead," chose to slay the dragon of . . . second-hand smoke.

It is not our intention to rehearse the evidence for and against second-hand smoke. Suffice to say that medical researchers are divided on the matter. Perhaps it poses some limited peril; perhaps not. But as we have seen, Dr. C. Everett Koop does not acknowledge shades of gray.

Casting caution and the scientific method to the wind, Koop included in the 1982 *Surgeon General's Report on Smoking and Health* a condemnation of what he termed "passive smoking" that was wholly unsupported by solid evidence. The phrase itself is a sterling example of Orwellian Newspeak. By "passive smoking" Koop did not mean a languid drag on a cigarette by a lotus-eating sybarite, half asleep, reclining on the couch, but rather the exposure to what is typically known as "second-hand smoke." (An even sillier term for it is "airborne cancer.") There is no such thing as "passive smoking"—either one smokes, which constitutes an action, or one is not smoking. Being in a room with one who is smoking cannot be called "smoking"—except, it seems, by government officials, who can by fiat change the very meaning of words, and quibble about even the definition of "is."

It must be noted that Koop was a pipe smoker until the 1970s.[31] Yes, the quidnunc who shamed his father into quitting smoking and who haughtily announced to his future wife that he could never marry her if she used the demon weed tobacco was himself a smoker during his married life. A grade-A hypocrite. Even worse—a creator of second-hand smoke. A facilitator of . . . *passive smoking*! An ignorer of no less than the 1964 report of . . . the Surgeon General!

In any event, Koop would later declare that second-hand smoke "causes many diseases, including cancer,"[32] a charge that no reputable researcher can make with certitude. In 1986 he issued the Surgeon General's *Health Consequences of Passive Smoking*, a farrago of unproven claims advertising themselves as Gospel Truth. What we have here is a man who mistakes his own biases and obsessions for truth; one name for such a person is "fanatic," though as we shall see in later chapters, whatever fanaticism Dr. Koop may possess has not gotten in the way of old-fashioned money grubbing.

Surgeon General Koop's war on smoking is revealing of both his character and ideology, so we shall examine it further. The first thing one notices, when combing through the record, is that Chick is not exactly a give-me-liberty-or-give-me-death kind of guy. His summation of the government's role in the war on tobacco is illustrative:

> [G]overnment has been important in both positive and negative ways. On the positive side, the government has raised excise and sales taxes on cigarettes, making cigarettes increasingly a painful pocketbook issue for smokers. Governments—federal, state, and local—have also severely restricted the areas where people can smoke in public. It is not legal to smoke on most public conveyances, in most retail stores, in virtually all government buildings, in all theaters and sports cen-

ters, and in many places where people work. A growing number of restaurants have either banned smoking or set aside nonsmoking areas.[33]

And so it goes. Every restriction on the action of free men and women is tallied on the positive side of the ledger. But we are a long way from paradise, in Koop's estimation. Federal taxes on cigarettes are too low. Tobacco is not sufficiently regulated by such agencies as the Food and Drug Administration. Vendors of these poisonous wares continue to exercise their First Amendment rights to advertise—and nothing drives Dr. Koop crazier than seeing an ad for a product of which he disapproves.

Questions of choice, of liberty, of the freedom to make decisions, never so much as furrow Koop's brow. He called for a ban on *all* cigarette advertising on billboards and in newspapers and magazines, dismissing the canard of free speech with the disturbingly authoritarian remark that "Free speech cannot injure the common welfare to serve the commercial interests of a few."[34] Which is to say that if you seek to vend something, you had best first get the permission of the rulers. This is not, to say the least, a classically American formulation.

Koop seems reduced to an almost sputtering rage when he contemplates the riches earned by tobacconists. The industry "flaunts its ability to buy its way into the marketplace of ideas and pollute it with its false and deadly information." It's odd to read an indictment of business for daring to promote its product and defend itself against attacks, but when Chick is in high dudgeon there's no stopping him. He huffed in indignation when representatives of tobacco companies sought to meet with him during his anti-smoking crusade. In full-dress righteousness, he denied that all the worldly riches the devil could offer would ever lead him to act as a shill: "No amount of money could ever entice me to represent a tobacco company under any circumstances."[35] How noble of him. A bit more than thirty pieces of silver *did* entice the good doctor to flack for killer diet drugs, though, as we shall detail in chapter 4.

Koop's account of his war on tobacco reads like a Puritan lady's tale of wandering into a brothel at orgy time. He is shocked, simply shocked, by its iniquity. At times, he fancies himself a gumshoe, a Philip Marlowe out to save the virtue of the helpless damsel America: "The deeper I probed into the murky, smoky world of tobacco power, the more I realized how extensive was the grasp of its tentacles."[36] He is hurrying, scurrying, hither and thither, rather like a . . . well, you know what, with its head cut off. He tries to browbeat the Pentagon into ending its practice of selling cheap cigarettes in military facilities. (The generals and admirals, evidently unimpressed by the Surgeon General's uniform, rebuff him.) He goes after smokeless tobacco—the chewing kind favored by so many generations of ballplayers. He somehow squeezes four questions about tobacco into the 1990 U.S. Census form, an intrusion that is nowhere authorized by the U.S. Constitution (as though that musty old document drafted by *smokers* and [gasp!] tobacco growers retains any relevance today!). When the quartet of queries is excised at the last minute, Koop blames "tobacco industry pressure"[37] instead of a rare fit of good sense by census drafters who had a qualm or two about sticking the Pinocchio-like snout of the federal government into the personal affairs of American citizens.

From time to time, Koop protested that he was "not advocating totalitarianism,"[38] a disavowal about as convincing as the collected sexual denials of Bill Clinton or Nixon's "I am not a crook" announcements. His "Smoke-Free Society—2000" initiative, launched in the fitting year of 1984, may as well have been titled "Liberty-Free Society—2000." Throughout, his actions were consistent with those of one who is dedicated to the erection of a Total State: he worked with the Coalition on Smoking OR Health to design a twelve-year curriculum of anti-smoking propaganda that could have come direct from the pages of Orwell or Huxley.

"[Y]ou have to get them while they're young," as Koop famously said, in a sentiment reminiscent of Ray Bradbury's *Fahrenheit 451*. Koop himself unintentionally illustrates the Chicken Little quality of his perpetual direness with his story of visiting an elementary school in Hawaii. The students had been indoctrinated only too well with the Smoke-Free Society—2000 catechism. "Who can tell me what's going to happen in the year 2000?" the Surgeon General asked the tykes. He called on a little boy in the back of the room.

"We are all going to die!"[39] the lad screamed.

Thus the triumph of Koopism. Unless we cede decisions over our own lives to credentialed experts and government officials, WE ARE ALL GOING TO DIE! (Never mind that we are all going to die anyway, and in any event, Dr. Koop will get rich beyond the dreams of most pediatric surgeons.)

Koop met resistance in his war on tobacco. Within a democratic republic, even one as malfunctioning as ours sometimes seems to be, those whom you are trying to punish or strip of liberty have the right to organize, the right to petition, the right to contest elections and legislative votes. So the last refuge of the prohibitionist scoundrel is usually medicine. Political issues, once medicalized, can be removed from the hurly-burly of the democratic process and placed upon a high shelf, accessible only to the muckamucks of the therapeutic state. So when Koop said that the issue is "not smoking, not tobacco, but nicotine addiction," or when he declaimed, absurdly, "Most smokers are drug addicts,"[40] he was seeking to circumvent the world of voters and legislators and cretins whose opinions differ from those of the good doctor. For once his propositions are accepted, the matter of smoking—or narcotic use, or eating fatty foods—can be removed from the political arena, where advocates of personal choice at least have a fighting chance, and placed under the vigilant eye of the Substance Abuse priesthood. Thus his proposal to de-politicize the job he once held: to vest the Surgeon General not only with greater coercive powers but also to insulate him from any pressure by elected officials.

"I think that the government has a perfect right to influence personal behavior to the best of its ability if it is for the welfare of the individual and the community as a whole,"[41] says Koop, complacent in the knowledge that he will be an influencer and you one of the vast herd of the influenced. The subordination of the individual to the "community as a whole" has a long and dishonorable lineage; how dispiriting—how chilling—that this totalitarian formula, the essential philosophy of communism, can be mouthed as just another platitude by the most powerful public-health official in the land of the free. Or free [*sic*], if Dr. Koop gets his way.

"If any other commonly consumed substance were labeled addictive, it would be taken off the shelves within a week,"[42] declares Koop, revealing his hand—enwrapped in the iron fist of Big Brotherism.

His jihad against the infidel cigarette won Koop fawning praise from the smokeless yuppies of the media. He found that "I had begun to earn back the credibility I had possessed in my previous surgical career."[43] The key, it seems, was to de-emphasize abortion, the issue he had ridden into the job, and play to the causes beloved of statist liberals. For if there is anything C. Everett Koop appears to love as much as instructing his inferiors in proper hygiene and body care, it is reading newspaper clips that lionize him, or seeing himself on television surrounded by famous people gazing at him with the look of blank adoration that Nancy Reagan used to shine upon her husband.

Once again, Koop drew an inappropriate lesson from his experience. After the smoking war, "I began to see the valuable ways in which the Surgeon General's position could be used to advance the health of the nation with moral suasion."[44] Ah, this is priceless. "Moral suasion." This term is generally understood to mean noncoercive persuasion. Just what is noncoercive about government-imposed advertising bans, higher taxes, and restrictions on smoking in every conceivable building or place other than the home (and they're getting to that, just you wait and see)? If this is moral suasion, one shudders to think what constitutes coercion in the mind of C. Everett Koop.

Koop the pipe-smoker declared war on other people's smokes. And he was no less the hypocrite when he joined an even older and more ignoble crusade: that of our grim neo-prohibitionists to virtually ban the advertisement, then the sale, and finally the consumption of alcohol.

Among other things, Chick Koop likes a drink now and then. Not just a glass of wine to wash down the soft cheeses at a Washington, DC soiree: no, Chick is a man's man, a virile, swaggering consumer of martinis. Emphasis on the plural, for most reports from friendly reporters of an evening at a fund-raiser with Dr. Koop mention, with evident surprise, that Koop is a martini drinker who stops at just one with as much difficulty as the proverbial Lay's potato chip eater. "After sipping his second Absolut vodka martini at Nantucket Cove on Thursday night, bearded and barrel-chested Dr. C. Everett Koop. . . "[45] began Jerry Berger in the *St. Louis Post-Dispatch*. Margaret Carlson of the suctorial *Time* swooned over "the 6–ft. 1–in., 210–lb. doctor, whose taste for red meat and martinis keeps him from losing his paunch. . . . "[46]

Far be it from the authors to malign a man for enjoying a martini or two (or three or . . .), but it does seem just the tiniest bit Pharisaical for the martini-guzzler to spend the nondrinking part of his day advocating a series of measures that might have come from the Women's Christian Temperance Union. "We couldn't have a better advocate than Everett Koop," gushed Christine Lubinski of the neo-prohibitionist National Council on Alcoholism—a group that regards Mothers Against Drunk Driving as sopping wets. Added Lubinski, using the Koopian tactic of medicalizing political issues, "We're not a bunch of moral crusaders trying to eliminate demon rum. This is a health movement, not a religious . . . moral movement."[47] So under the mask of medicine, Surgeon General Koop and his yuppie Carrie Nation comrades excise those liberties that they find offensive. The blue-ribbon report, they have found, is mightier than the hatchet.

In his final Surgeon General's report, Koop took aim—ostensibly—at drunk driving. But there was more to it than that. No one this side of the handful of geriatric members of the Foster Brooks Fan Club still extant defends drunks behind the wheels of automobiles. Yet Koop's recommendations targeted the *legal* drinker, even though the Eighteenth Amendment was repealed in 1933, however much to the chagrin of the National Council on Alcoholism.

For instance, Koop demanded that the federal government force the states to slash the permissible blood alcohol concentration (BAC) of drivers to a minuscule 0.04 percent. A sip from a second martini thus would turn many of us into "drunk" drivers—but then laws are made for mere mortals, not for the likes of C. Everett Koop, who seems never to include himself among the masses to whom his strictures would apply.

The martini-swilling Surgeon General also called for steep increases in the excise taxes on beer, wine, and distilled spirits; for mandatory blood alcohol tests whenever any driver in America is injured in an automobile accident; for increased federal subsidies for televised anti-alcohol propaganda ("pro-health and pro-safety messages"[48]); and restricting alcohol advertising, including that at rock concerts and sporting events. Koop conceded the lack of direct scientific evidence that advertising boosts consumption, but why scuttle such a magnificent project as prohibition just because a few numbers don't add up? After leaving office, Koop shed whatever inhibitions he once had and called for a total ban on alcohol advertising, leading New York University law professor Burt Neuborne, former legal director of the American Civil Liberties Union, to protest the Koop plan as "a mortal blow to the fundamental moral, political, social and economic structure of America."[49] The grandiosity of the phrasing no doubt pleased Koop.

No avenue of human enjoyment was too small to escape the meddling of Koop; he even called for abolishing the Happy Hour. Ronald R. Rumbaugh, president of the National Beer Wholesalers Association, charged that "drunk driving was a mere pretext for a general attack on alcohol consumption that rivals anything we've seen since Prohibition."[50] (Amusingly, the foremost congressional Koopian was

Rep. Joseph Kennedy [D-MA], grandson of a surpassingly vulgar bootlegger. But then young Joe was widely regarded as the dumbest member of the House—a distinction since inherited by his cousin Patrick [D-MA]. Whatever Dr. Koop is, he is not dumb.)

Striding ever more purposefully in his vice admiral's uniform, Surgeon General Koop set out for territories uncharted. "Some of the things that I had in mind were issues usually beyond the purview of the Surgeon General,"[51] said Koop. He can say that again.

Koop's agenda was moral, not bureaucratic, reform.

Those who had made possible his elevation to the Celebrity Nation—Senator Helms and the pro-life crowd—were deeply disappointed by his tenure. He largely ignored abortion, knowing on which side the bread of good publicity is buttered, until late in President Reagan's second term, when he sent the President a letter stating that the effects of abortion on the health (particularly the mental health) of women who have abortions are unclear. "I have concluded in my review of this issue that, at this time, the available scientific evidence about the psychological sequalae of abortion simply cannot support either the preconceived beliefs of those pro-life or of those pro-choice people," wrote Koop.[52]

This does not appear to be an untruth, but it is passing strange: scant evidence did not constrain the crusading Surgeon General when it came to such dubious hazards as second-hand smoke. And the Koop letter would come to haunt those who had been his strongest supporters when he had needed them most: as Gregg L. Cunningham of the Center for Bio-Ethical Reform wrote Koop in 1993, "it has been my painful experience to have been repeatedly assaulted by abortion advocates who gleefully beat me over the head with your now infamous report to President Reagan discrediting clinical studies purporting to link abortion with adverse psychological reactions."[53]

Koop sought to reinvigorate the morale of the Public Health Service's Commissioned Corps: 6,200 doctors strong and often a bit down at the mouth, used as they were to the usual slights about the inferiority of "government doctors." For years, budget-cutters had had the Commissioned Corps in their sights: at enormous expense, the Corps provided health care that could be provided at less expense—and perhaps greater skill—by others. Koop contemptuously cited a Reagan administration official who wondered why the PHS Commissioned Corps had to service the Merchant Marine: "Why don't all those Merchant Mariners have Blue Cross-Blue Shield like the rest of us?"[54] To Koop, the question was absurd; to "the rest of us," well, why not?

And so Koop, when not upbraiding the citizenry for drinking or smoking or eating foods of which he disapproved, played the old bureaucratic game of protecting his bailiwick. Whatever parsimonious impulses Ronald Reagan had were not shared by his Surgeon General. Koop fought off cuts to the PHS—heaven forfend that the employees of the National Oceanographic and Atmospheric Administration should have their cholesterol levels tested by other than Koop's Commissioned Corps. Koop is credited for revitalizing the Corps not by streamlining it, or attracting higher quality doctors, but by saving it from the budget-cutter's knife and . . . by making its members wear their uniforms! This was a bitter pill for some PHS doctors, who had joined in the 1960s and early 1970s to avoid Vietnam and the whole military culture, but they soon learned that to C. Everett Koop, the uniform made—in many ways was more important than—the man.

For five-and-a-half years Koop studiously and very conspicuously avoided any mention of the acronym AIDS. He blamed the Reagan administration for silencing him, though to all appearances his mouth bore no muzzle. Rather, his own cowardice stilled his tongue: he dared not speak lest he not be reappointed to the post he had come to cherish. For there are few persons less newsworthy than an ex-Surgeon General.

When Koop finally did come out—his tongue, and that of others in the administration, loosed by the death of Reagan friend Rock Hudson from AIDS—it was with a vengeance. Whereas before he had trembled even to name the malady, now he insisted that the merest prepubescent children should be instructed in matters sexual in the public schools. "Sex education should begin at the earliest age possible," he harrumphed, and when pressed for specificity, he allowed that the third grade seemed about right.[55] He applied $20 million of taxpayers' monies to launch a truly immense mailing of 107 million letters about AIDS to the nation's households. His office published *The Surgeon General's Report on Acquired Immune Deficiency Syndrome,* and he later voiced astonishment that President Reagan had not actually read the report—as though any president, let alone one with as un-voracious a reading appetite as Reagan, reads every piece of paper disgorged by his bureaucracy. He boasted that he had used "such words as 'penis,' 'vagina,' [and] 'condom'"[56]—a regular Henry Miller of the bureaucracy. Never mind that Miller was an anarchist who'd have been appalled to see the federal government stuffing people's mailboxes with its propaganda, for whatever cause. (To be fair, AIDS elicited from Koop his only known acknowledgement of constitutional liberties: he quite rightly opposed mandatory testing of American citizens for the AIDS virus.)

"[S]uddenly I found myself praised by my former liberal adversaries and condemned by my former conservative allies,"[57] he marveled. Koop's response was to soak in the honeyed words of adulation while demonizing his critics: those with the temerity to disagree were "crazies," "misinformed, misguided or vindictive" victims of a "strange mentality." Rather than credit those who had differing opinions with sense and intelligence, he scoffed that they were in thrall to "old fears and prejudices."[58] He refused to see that federally prescribed sex education for eight-year-olds might be an affront to those families who prefer to teach morality within the home. Koop's righteousness was by now nigh intolerable: it was impossible to dissent from his *ex cathedra* pronouncements without being a benighted member of the legion of darkness. When an old ally in the right-to-life cause later took him to task for failing to object to the abortion-coverage provisions in the ill-fated, if Koop-supported, Clinton health care proposal, Koop huffed, "I am responsible not to you but to God for the way I act."[59] (An unkind critic might take this as a declaration that he is responsible only to himself.) "You are mean spirited, Mr. Cunningham," Koop concluded his letter to a gentleman who had written what was actually a rather polite, if critical, letter. But "mean spirited" is one of those empty phrases employed by the Ins to silence the Outs. And C. Everett Koop has become about as In as one can be.

What price glory? Tens of thousands of Americans would die of AIDS-related complications in a near-epidemic sedulously ignored by the Surgeon General, but once he found his voice Koop rose ever upward into the empyrean of the famous. The breathless jottings in his 1987 diary are revealing: "Went on ABC. . . . Appeared on PBS. . . . Had lunch with George Bush. . . . Taped a good Public Broadcasting System show on AIDS with Susan Dey of *L.A. Law*. . . . Breakfast with Morgan Fairchild."[60]

You get the idea. Chick was Important. He hung around with Celebrities. Taping shows with the good-looking daughter from *The Partridge Family*. And Morgan Fairchild. For *breakfast*, for goodness sake! Oo-la-la!

But all good things must end, and C. Everett Koop's stay as Surgeon General was about up. A Surgeon General serves a four-year term, not necessarily conterminous with that of the president. Because of his long confirmation fight, Koop's second term spilled into the early months of the Bush administration. Would new President Bush keep him? The suspense was killing Koop, despite his studied nonchalance. He lobbied hard for a reappointment, but by this time his name was in such bad odor among conservative Republicans that George Bush declined to accede to Koop's request to stay on. Bush was, in effect, throwing a sop to the religious right, which had come to loathe its former pet for his volubility on the matter of AIDS. So C. Everett Koop lost his job in a symbolic act—just as he had "earned" his job. He who lives by the sop dies by the sop.

Koop's account of the Bush decision reveals the extent to which his sanctimony and self-regard had exceeded all human limits. He concedes that he did lobby for reappointment, just a wee little bit, but his real desire was a promotion to Secretary of Health and Human Services. He hadn't a chance in hell of getting HHS, but Koop says that the day after Bush nominated Dr. Louis Sullivan to that post the magnanimous Chick called Sullivan's office and left the message "that of all the people who were standing in line to advise him, I was the one who had no personal agenda, no axe to grind."[61] (Perhaps because the axes were already in the backs of the alcohol and tobacco industries and his erstwhile right-to-life friends.) Then, to top it off, that ingrate Dr. Sullivan did not return the Mighty Koop's call: the nerve! The gall! Surely this man was in the pocket of the ______ (choose your favorite poison) lobby.

Thus C. Everett Koop returned to private life. Or did he? For he had gotten an (unfortunately legal) rush from years of wielding the cudgel of state. By the time George Bush sent him packing, "I began to feel like the Surgeon General of all the people. . . . I had become family doctor to the nation."[62] An alienist might diagnose this as megalomania. Alas, there was no cure. For over the next decade the former Surgeon General would do his level best to make himself doctor not to separate families, with their variety and idiosyncrasy, but doctor to what he imagined to be the family of America: a herd of ignorant cattle who respond best to the prod. He had learned, he said, that "the moralist and the scientist could walk hand in hand"[63]—leading the rest of us hellward, into the fool's perdition of closely regulated lives.

He would also make himself a pile of money. He became rich, not by curing the sick or inventing techniques and technologies that enable others to heal the ailing, but by selling his name as a harlot vends her virtue. "I was not about to sell or rent my integrity and the public trust,"[64] Koop declared righteously after he left office. He boasted of turning down endorsement opportunities for cereals and condoms—but within a short time he would be shilling for far more dubious products.

C. Everett Koop wanted to take the position of Surgeon General where no man or woman had gone before. He did. He made it the most annoying office in government, and a springboard to wealth for whoever can wear convincingly the harlequin's uniform.

So little time, so many vices to outlaw, so much money to make running the old Integrity scam. Upon stepping down from his Surgeon General post Koop ran around frantically, mouthing off about everything and everybody, as though he feared his newsworthiness was about up and he wanted to squeeze out every last headline and buck he could.

One day he might be calling for a "total ban"[65] on alcohol advertising. (Perhaps then the sales of beer would be as pathetic as the sales of the C. Everett Koop home health-care tapes pushed by Time-Life.) "Alcohol is a toxic, potentially addictive drug and the greatest killer of American young people," he declared—presumably not whilst slurping his second martini—in 1992. "If alcohol and tobacco were now for the first time being tested for popular consumption, the regulatory agencies we entrust with watching out for our health would disallow their use."[66] No doubt the doctor slept off his martini buzz that night dreaming prohibitionist dreams. Another day he was urging mandatory bike helmet laws as chairman of the National Safe Kids Campaign—one of those ingeniously named crusades, for who can possibly be against safe kids? When not issuing pontifical bulls from his Bethesda, Maryland, office, just outside Washington, D.C., he was flying to Washington State to campaign for gun control. His press coverage was even more fawning than when he had worn the uniform, if that is possible: "[H]e is widely recognized as the nation's foremost fighter for public health,"[67] purled a typical puff piece. (Substitute "his own wallet" for "public health" and you've hit the bull's-eye.)

His speaking fee was in the range of $25,000, or about the going rate for an ex-president. (Then again, the compelling oratory of Gerald Ford and Jimmy Carter are perhaps not fair yardsticks.) Yet by playing up the occasional freebie, Koop kept his press clippings warm and fuzzy. For instance, he made a pair of public service announcements promoting the use of animals in medical research for the Foundation for Biomedical Research, on whose pharmaceutical-funded board he served. Adweek's *Marketing Week* explained Koop's waiver of a fee as part and parcel of his principled refusal "to cash in on his visibility the way other Reagan officials had."[68] (The director of the Koop PSAs, Barry Seidman, noted that crew members were terrified to smoke in front of Dr. Koop. "During breaks to reload," Seidman said, "smokers would take off into the back room. It was like the smoky high-school bathroom."[69])

He picked up the Albert Schweitzer Prize for Humanitarianism in Baltimore, pocketing $10,000. (Humanitarianism pays a lot better today than in the dark old days of St. Francis of Assisi.) He won an Emmy. He was awarded—but, strangely, did not show up to accept—the Senior Coalition's "Finger of Shame" award for his flacking on behalf of Glaxo-Wellcome. President Clinton awarded him a Presidential Medal of Freedom, the highest honor conferred by the U.S. government upon civilians, for "putting sound medical advice ahead of ideology,"[70] as, presumably, when he supported the Clinton's nationalized health care plan.

The enlistment of Dr. Koop in the various health crusades (nonvenereal department) of the Clinton administration began early, with the ill-fated 1993 Hillary health care plan that almost sunk the administration before it got out of port. Koop was still bitter that George Bush had inexplicably ignored his conspicuous talents and given the job of HHS Secretary to that old nonentity Dr. Louis Sullivan. And then Sullivan had the nerve not to return Chick's call. Such temerity would not go unpunished!

The Clintons knew just how to stroke Koop. Hillary praised him as "thoughtful, courageous, and independent,"[71] whereupon he forfeited that vaunted independence and went on the road, plumping for the Clinton plan. He accepted an assignment to whip up support for Clinton Care among physicians—not an easy task, given that he had frequently been critical of physicians when they, well, disagreed with the pronunciamentos of Dr. C. Everett Koop. And in fact the good doctor failed miserably at this job, as doctors outside the federal bureaucracy displayed a notable lack of enthusiasm for Clinton Care. His other job was to "signal to [Republicans] it's OK to support Clinton's reforms"[72]—a botched assignment on the order of delegating Hugh Hefner to inform a nubile starlet's parents that their daughter is doing just fine and not to worry. If there was one Reagan official whom Republicans had learned not to trust, it was the one who was so lovingly coddled by the press—the one who had refused to cash in, etc., etc.

The health care plan fiasco was not without its lighter side, as Koop revealed an almost staggering incomprehension of basic American principles. He proposed, for example, that we ought to have a national debate on the question, "Does the Constitution or the Bill of Rights provide the right to health care?" (To forestall a multibillion dollar "national dialogue" of the sort beloved by the Clintons, we'll give a simple and comprehensive answer: No.) Koop the philosopher-king was also given to musing on such bizarre matters as the meaning of the "pursuit of liberty." In the first place, Mr. Jefferson and the signers of the Declaration of Independence counted "liberty," not the pursuit thereof, as an inalienable right. But given Koop's chariness of liberty, perhaps the significance of his New and Improved version of the Declaration is the fact that not everything that is pursued is caught, and wouldn't it be wonderful for the public health tyrants if liberty eluded capture? In any event, Koop asked if by the "pursuit of liberty" the Founders meant that the state should provide "a hip replacement for everybody regardless of age, regardless of ability to use the new gadget?"[73] If we may again be permitted to bring this line of speculation to a merciful close . . . No.

Koop summed up his ideal of governance in a 1992 interview with *Business & Health.* Asked about health care reform, he replied, "I think we can have a better system, but it can come only from the top." Dropping, for a moment, the imagery of war, he switched to the language of its sporting substitute, football. "I have one theme that I keep coming back to: You've got to have somebody who is calling the shots, who can say to all the players: 'When I snap the ball, this is where I want you to go.'"[74] Okay, so he seems to be talking about a center rather than a quarterback, but you get the picture. Koop, by the way, did play football, at least for a few blinks of the eye, at Dartmouth. His position—center. So perhaps the "When I snap the ball" phrase wasn't a flub after all. For years Koop has wowed the rubber chicken circuit with his story of the almost incredible insensitivity of Dartmouth's legendary coach, Earl "Red" Blaik. In this tale—how tall only the indomitable Chick knows—Blaik is bowled over by the sight of a green freshman stud practicing the interception of the ball.

"What's your name?" asked the grizzled coach.

"Chick Koop," chirps the lad.

"Do you know you run like Buckler?" says the coach, talking the way football coaches always talk in movies. "I haven't seen anybody run like that since I left the [West] Point."

A star is born—but snuffed out oh so soon. For at a subsequent practice this proto-Butkus named Koop makes a spectacular interception and is running to daylight when a "vicious" tackle by not one—did you really think a single Dartmouth boy could pull down Koop?—but two players knocks the star out cold. When he comes to he has double vision, and it does not go away. Several days later, Koop visits Professor Bielschowsky, "the most knowledgeable person in the world at that time regarding the function of the extraocular muscles of the eye." (You didn't think he'd just drop into Sterling Vision Center to be seen by an ophthamological plebe, do you?) Dr. Bielschowsky asked the injured center his major. "Premed," replied the ex-vivisectionist. "Let me see your hands," demanded the doctor, who surveys Koop's mitts with intensity.

"They're beautiful," coos the doctor. "They're surgeon's hands. So you not only risk your sight and maybe your life, but your hands and your career. Such foolishness."

Well, what was Koop to do? The world's expert in the function of the extraocular muscles of the eye had spoken, and insisted that for the sake of humanity, not to mention the life of one C. Everett Koop, the center resign from the team. Surely Coach Blaik would understand.

Surely Coach Blaik did not understand. "So, in other words, you're a coward,"[75] he told Koop—in Koop's telling. Thereafter the coaches and athletes, his former teammates, shunned him. They would rather he go blind, die, deprive the world of such beautiful hands, all for the sake of a dumb game.

Or at least that is C. Everett Koop's version. One wonders how—or if—Red Blaik would remember the tale, were he still around. But he is not, and his purpose in death is to be just another tile in the mosaic of the Koop Legend.

But we digress. The subject was Koop's cooptation by the Clintons. "Without a single law, a single regulation, he has done more for health care reform in the past four months than all of his living predecessors put together,"[76] gushed Koop of the President in September 1993. But Clinton's Rube Goldberg scheme never got off the ground, and by mid-1994 you didn't need a weatherman to tell you that it would be stuck forever in the doldrums. So Dr. Koop took a step back; by May 1994, he was allowing as how the President's plan was "better than any of the other current plans,"[77] but that it wasn't quite what he had in mind. A bit too bureaucratic, he thought, and incomplete as well, what with its shocking absence of new taxes on beer, wine, liquor, ammunition, and handguns. Not that he wanted healthcare to "be treated like any other business, as an opportunity for investors to make money," he said in pooh-poohing managed care, under which "[p]rofit, not health, is the prime objective."[78]

Through it all, though, he remained faithful to Mrs. Clinton. (And what a novel experience that must have been for her.) "Not only is she well versed in the subject, but she comes through as a compassionate person who wants to learn more, who is very flexible. . . . When I come away from a forum with her, I feel that we've accomplished our purpose."[79] In June 1994 Mrs. Clinton would receive the American Diabetes Association's C. Everett Koop Medal for "excellence in wellness promotion and disease prevention." In 1996, at the White House signing ceremony for one of those picayune laws upon which President Clinton sought to build his legacy before he discovered the joys of war, Dr. Koop sat in the front row with Hillary Rodham Clinton. They were thick as thieves, and their bond would only be strengthened during the Clinton administration's puritanical crusade against that ogre to top all ogres: Big Tobacco. (Or, in practice, little cigarette smokers.)

Koop's assistance cannot be said to have boosted the fortunes of Clintonian legislation, whether in the tobacco fields or the thicket of health care. But it was public, it was vocal, and you had better believe there was payback.

Lest the naive think that Koop's ultimately ineffective support came without a price, five years after the health care plan's messy birth, enterprising reporters broke the story that on the very day that Koop met with Clinton to "discuss the health care plan,"[80] the Clinton administration overrode the objections of military officials and granted a waiver permitting C. Everett Koop to be buried among the 250,000 veterans, presidents, and their families at Arlington National Cemetery. Koop had always been one of those non-soldiers who gets weak-kneed at the sight of a man in a uniform; the fact that he did not serve in the Second World War obviously bothered him, for he wasted few opportunities to assert, without much documentation, that he had been declared "essential" to the war effort. It was the old "I can do more on the home front" routine, which is sometimes true, and as long as the braggart isn't too loud, most of us don't bother to object. But Koop has also used the language of militarism to explain his politics: he's always agitating for a declaration of war on something or other, whether fat or tobacco or AIDS or kids who don't wear bike helmets, and so it was no big surprise that he lobbied his way into the largest and most revered veterans' cemetery in the country.

But then someone turned the heat up, and it was sexton, spare that dirt. For late in 1997, it was revealed that the Clinton administration had been granting an unprecedented number of waivers allowing normally ineligible persons to be interred in our nation's most hallowed burial ground. Among the most notorious was a sleazy Democratic fund-raiser and ambassador named Larry Lawrence, whose remains were disinterred from Arlington and reburied in San Diego when it was learned that he had lied about service in the merchant marine.

Until 1967, any honorably discharged veteran was eligible for burial at Arlington. But veterans of the Second World War began dying, and with no end in sight for the Vietnam War, administrators feared that the cemetery might soon be full. (As it is, the Army estimates that the 70,000 unused grave sites will be occupied by 2025.) A list of burial rules were drawn up: rules that would bar C. Everett Koop from spending eternity in Arlington, just as the pre-1967 rules would have done. After all, he was not a veteran, however much he enjoyed preening in his Surgeon General's costume.

Yet in August 1994 President Clinton informed the Army that "Koop had been granted an exemption from the rules, a promise virtually never made to a living person,"[81] according to the *Washington Post*. In fact, promising a living and noneligible person that he will be buried at Arlington was "unprecedented,"[82] said Rep. Terry Everett (R-AL), chairman of the House Veterans Committee. The General Accounting Office, asked to investigate the trading of burial sites for cash and lobbying help, determined that the Koop waiver request was routed through two typical avenues—the White House chief of staff and counsel—and one not so typical: the office of the First Lady. "I do everything Dr. Koop tells me to do," Hillary had said upon the launching of Shape Up, America!—apparently her assistance even extended unto death.

Outraged Republicans vowed to tighten the rules for burial at Arlington. Senator Chuck Hagel (R-NE), a veteran who was wounded in Vietnam, said of the link between Koop's lobbying and his posthumous real estate arrangement, "It is far more serious than just an implied deal. What we're talking about here is giving sacred resting spots of our nation's veterans away as deals, as rewards, as bargaining chips . . . and quid pro quo."[83]

The heat became so intense that Dr. Koop acted in a most un-Koopian fashion: he backed down. On February 4, 1998, he announced that "I hereby relinquish any claim to burial in Arlington Cemetery." But far be it from America's Family Physician to leave it at that. Rather than slink away, shame-faced, as a man with a normal sense of humility would, Koop magnanimously declared that he was giving up the ghost-box "without rancor"[84]—a classic Clintonian formulation, really, in which the wrongdoer forgives those he has harmed or offended.

The Koop arrogance was also at full throttle when in 1998 a coalition of Clintonian liberals and yuppie Republicans declared war—CEK's favorite metaphor—on that venerable vice of the working class, cigarette smoking. They did not phrase it that way, of course: no sense letting tens of millions of Americans—more pertinently, voters—know that you've got them in your sights. No, the putative enemy was Big Tobacco. The means of waging this war was a negotiated settlement between the attorneys general of the states and the big, bad tobacco industry. Now, "negotiated" does not quite capture the nature of the settlement, for it was "negotiated" in the sense that one negotiates with a mugger who has put a gun to your head and requested a donation from your wallet to his.

Koop roamed far and wide, instructing benighted state legislatures as to just what they should do with their share of the swag. In Minnesota, where the driving force behind the tobacco shakedown was has-been political son Hubert Humphrey III, the attorney general who lost the 1998 governor's race to the former professional wrestler, Jesse "The Body" Ventura, Koop and his comrade-in-coercion David Kessler, former director of the U.S. Food and Drug Administration, were named to head the Minnesota Partnership for Action Against Tobacco, which pocketed $202 million to fund its busybody activities. The ex-Surgeon General was then off to Hawaii—where, if you will recall, he had once convinced children that they were all gonna die. Speculating—or should we say fessing up to the real substance of his dreams—Koop told the islanders that if he were "king, czar or dictator of Hawaii,"[85] he would spend every last penny of the $1.2 billion windfall from the tobacco settlement on anti-smoking propaganda. (Small-minded legislators had actually considered using it to close the budget deficit.) He also found time to campaign in California for Proposition 10, an initiative to place a fifty cents-a-pack tax on cigarettes in order to fund a variety of welfare-state programs. The initiative was chaired by Rob Reiner, the middlebrow movie director best known for playing the torpid liberal "Meathead" on *All in the Family.*

Koop's loathing of the demon weed knew no bounds: Koop called on consumers to boycott Kraft and Nabisco foods in order to punish their corporate parents, tobacco giants Philip Morris and R. J. Reynolds. The ex-Surgeon General had met the enemy, and it looked a lot like those blue-and-white macaroni-and-cheese boxes. He also chastised American companies for selling cigarettes abroad, in a shocking display of free enterprise. Foreigners, it seems, are easy marks, for "these countries lack a Surgeon General's warning on tobacco."[86] Ain't we lucky to be livin' in America!

All this was too much even for so moderate a politician as the late-model Bob Dole, who by his hapless 1996 presidential campaign had been reduced to the sort of mush that the earlier Dole would have eaten for breakfast. Interviewed by the annoyingly perky yuppie Katie Couric on NBC's "Today" show, Dole opined that Koop had become an anti-tobacco fanatic because he "watches the liberal media and he probably got carried away."

"He's brainwashed?" sneered Couric.

"Probably, a little bit,"[87] replied Dole, sending the networks and major papers into conniption fits in defense of the sainted Dr. Koop—"America's bearded icon of solicitous medical integrity,"[88] in the fatuous phrase of the *Washington Post's* Mary McGrory. (McGrory, who churned out sententious nonsense like McDonald's makes hamburgers, was the woman who said after JFK's death that "we'll never laugh again." More accurately, she might have predicted that no one would ever read her column with a straight face again.)

Koop's zealousness helped torpedo the larger tobacco settlement, however, which the opportunistic Senator John McCain (R-AZ) had painstakingly crafted. In the midst of extraordinary tax increases and various punitive measures visited upon the satanic Big Tobacco, McCain had included legal protections for the industry—protections that would keep it from being sued out of existence by ravenous lawyers. At the insistence of Koop and Kessler, who became the Dour Duo of the Neo-Prohibitionist Bloc in the Senate, these safeguards were stripped from the bill, for as Koop thundered, "I see no reason we should agree to anything that grants this rogue industry any form of immunity or liability protection."[89]

That Koop was not an elected member of the U.S. Senate—part of the "we" who decides what should or should not be included in a bill—seems to have slipped his no-doubt overstimulated mind. In fact, such notorious tools of Big Tobacco as the American Cancer Society, the American Heart Association, and the National Center for Tobacco-Free Kids publicly broke with Koop in endorsing the principle of limited liability. But Chick was unmovable: the tobacco industry must be destroyed. And so McCain's bill, backed by Clinton, died.

Former Clinton guru Dick Morris, the toe-sucking political soothsayer, blamed the McCain bill's death on the "greed" and "unbridled arrogance"[90] of Koop and Kessler. Not only did they make plain that their intention was the destruction of an industry that employs hundreds of thousands of Americans, Koop also professed to feeling "shame"[91] at being a Republican: the party not of Lincoln but of nicotine, or so Koop seemed to believe. This was not the sort of remark to endear Koop to his old party. The days when the Clintonites might send Dr. Koop out as an emissary to the GOP were long gone.

But the capstone of Koopian Arrogance—an act that even his closest allies rolled their eyes over—came in March 1998. A House subcommittee invited Koop and Kessler to testify on the proposed tobacco settlement. They refused. And just why did they refuse? Because they would not agree to be sworn in. You see, five tobacco executives had testified two months earlier, and for Koop and Kessler to actually take oaths would place them "on some sort of parity" with these vile tobacco beasts. In a letter to the subcommittee chairman, Koop and Kessler wrote, "We have each devoted much of our professional careers to . . . working for the public health. We see no reason for the committee to suggest that our testimony about tobacco now requires that we be . . . treated akin to tobacco executives."[92]

Well!!! The subcommittee staff informed the Sanctimonious K's that "high-level witnesses" are routinely sworn in, but to no avail. They would not swear to tell the truth. And given Dr. Koop's habit of making broad assertions based on the narrowest evidence—and given his newfound fortune, his increasingly intimate ties with . . . business executives! . . . and his role as shill for the diet industry, which has aspects so sinister it can make the tobacco boys look like a kids' lemonade stand, perhaps it was for the best that Dr. Koop did not pledge to tell the truth. For the truth about Koop bears little resemblance to the flattering portraits drawn by his acolytes and camp followers.

2

Big Bellies, Fat Heads: The Sick Obsession with Weight

"The trouble is that bouncing, fat babies are considered beautiful."[1]

—C. Everett Koop

"[W]e calculate that by the year 2230, 100% of adults in the USA will be overweight . . . "[2]

—John Foreyt and Ken Goodrick, *The Lancet*

The First Nag was not to go gently into the good night of retirement. He was, rather, to follow the road to riches, a road paved with greed, avarice, and cupidity. It was the gold brick road which he had criticized so often in his role as the Conscience of American Medicine. Koop had denounced "doctors and hospitals who succumb to the temptation of greed." He pointed to polls showing that 40 percent of medical students say they chose medicine "because it's a way to make a comfortable living."[3] Well, the living that former Surgeon General Koop made was more than comfortable—and it was made possible, in part, by one of our age's great perversions: the physically and emotionally unhealthy mania for dieting.

Ahead, in the distance, two paths converge: the money trail down which Dr. Koop so purposefully strode, and the avenue of emaciation followed by so many unfortunates, mostly women, who have been sold a dangerous bill of goods by the elephantine diet industry and its shills (including one C.E.K.). There is sickness, even death at this convergence—as well as a handsome profit for the imposing man with the stern visage and Old Testament beard.

On paper, C. Everett Koop was not the ideal candidate to lead an anti-fat jihad. He weighs in at 210 pounds and regularly feasts on red meat, french fries, deviled eggs, potato chips, cheeseburgers, and honey-roasted peanuts. These are among his good qualities, yet they are not the sort usually found in hairshirt-wearing, bean-eating Fitness Nannies. But just as downing a few martinis didn't keep Koop out of the neo-prohibitionist corner, nor does his taste for grease and fat disqualify him from the leading role in the you'd-better-do-what-we-say-if-you-know-what's-good-for-you-sounding organization Shape Up America! "For myself, I'm counting on my genes," Koop has said when asked about his non-monkish eating habits. "If your cholesterol is okay and you think your genes are good, why should you sit on a hill the rest of your life and eat yogurt?"[4]

"Nobody loves a fat man," lamented Fatty Arbuckle in the silent movie *The Round-Up*. Least of all those who seek to fatten their bank accounts by browbeating him into potentially life-threatening slimness.

Unfortunately, Arbuckle's plaint has become widely accepted. (In the actor's case, it would have been more accurate to say that nobody loves a debauched fat man who rapes a girl with a foreign object and accidentally kills her. One doubts that anyone would love a thin man who did such a thing either.) In any event, perhaps 40 percent of women and 24 percent of men are dieting or otherwise trying to shed pounds at any moment in America.[5] (The numbers rise in the early fall, as dieters swell with resolve, and fall around Christmas time, when the secular symbol of the season is a fat man whom everybody loves.) An additional 25 to 30 percent are trying to maintain their current weight. An absurd 74 percent of Americans "admit" that they need to lose weight.[6]

Public opinion surveys on matters of weight, if not weighty matters, are mind-boggling. One 1985 poll found that 90 percent of Americans think that we weigh too much. In a 1988 survey of University of Michigan freshmen, just 15 percent were satisfied with their weight.[7] A 1984 *Glamour* magazine survey of 33,000 women revealed that three-fourths believed themselves too fat. (This was not a sample of hefty women; only a quarter were overweight using the slender-happy standards of the Metropolitan Life Insurance Company.)

Americans spend about one billion dollars each year on the multimedia freak show of diet books, videos, and tapes. (Instead of listening to this tripe while you drive, why not walk to your destination? And when you return, congratulate yourself with a glass of wine—very heart-smart, as they say—and a protein-and-iron-rich hamburger topped with a prostate-cancer-fighting tomato.) They fork over closer to two billion dollars annually to the Jenny Craigs and other commercial weight-loss centers. This money isn't coming from the chronically fat; John LaRosa of Marketdata Enterprises, who tracks the diet business, says, "The big money in the industry is for cosmetic weight loss of 10 to 20 pounds."[8]

The diet merchants, armed with their government health guidelines and with C. Everett Koop firmly planted in their hip pocket, prey upon the lost, the gullible, and the melancholy chunky to the tune of up to $50 billion a year, or so estimates the U.S. Center for Health Statistics.

We say "prey upon" not out of any animus toward business—indeed, the authors are economists of a decidedly free-market bent—but because this industry feeds upon superstition and fear. According to the Centers for Disease Control, an astounding 62 percent of those women and 44 percent of those men who are dieting at any given time *are not overweight*, even by the federal government's overly strict standards.[9] The more realistic National Task Force on the Prevention and Treatment of Obesity calculated that only one in eight Americans is overweight.

Most remarkably—and dispiritingly—this diet industry boom has come despite the fact that the current assessment of the effectiveness of weight-loss programs has changed very little since pioneer researcher Dr. Albert Stunkard of the University of Pennsylvania declared in 1958, "Most obese persons will not stay in treatment for obesity. Of those who stay in treatment, most will not lose weight, and of those who do lose weight, most will regain it."[10] And today? As dietitian Elizabeth Ward, spokeswoman for the American Dietetic Association, says, "Many people who come to see me for help have gone through every single one of the commercial diet programs first."[11] Their wallets are lighter—a typical four-month stint in a commercial diet program costs in the neighborhood of $700—but the hips on which the wallet sit are no smaller.

Poundage, which had always been associated with prosperity, is now linked with gluttony. "It is a problem,"[12] frets Dr. Xavier Pi-Sunyer, chairman of the National Heart, Lung and Blood Institute task force of the National Institutes of Health—and the father of the controversial new Body Mass Index (BMI) guidelines. "We're the fattest nation in the world." So we are supposed to wail and gnash teeth over the fact that the average weight of American men and women (given a height of 5'4") is 162 lbs., which exceeds the average of Southern Europeans (156 lbs.), Eastern Europeans (150 lbs.), Western and Central Europeans (147 lbs.), Northern Europeans (146 lbs.), South and Central Americans (145 lbs.), Africans (137 lbs.), and Asians (128 lbs.) Might this in fact be cause for rejoicing? Isn't a rounded figure or prosperous gut a sign of wealth?

Not on your life. Every pound above some mythical mean bears the mark of the devil. Even chubby infants are cause not for rejoicing but bemoaning, for as Dr. Koop dolefully lectures, "The trouble is that bouncing, fat babies are considered beautiful. But fat babies become fat kids; fat kids become fat adolescents, and fat adolescents become fat adults."[13]

The villains are sometimes ludicrous in this white hat-black hat morality play—and we should point out that the black hat is often worn by an American with black skin, for African-Americans are disproportionately represented in the "overweight category," which brands them with the mark of Cain in the minds of the nutrition zealots. One of the silliest evils is "portion distortion," much lamented by the fatophobes: that is, businesses are flayed for serving us *too much food for our money!* What's wrong with these cruel capitalists anyway? Don't they know that the U.S. government defines a single serving of french fries as consisting of a grand total of 10 of those golden slices? A carton at a fast-food joint may contain 25, 30, even 40 individual fries. They're killing us with their kindness!

"Restaurant portions are very much out of control,"[14] one nutrition consultant complained to the *Washington Post*. Store-bought muffins sometimes tip the scales at eight ounces—six and one-half ounces more than the U.S. government says a muffin should weigh. This is so insidious that the tobacco industry must be involved somehow.

Our ancestors would find this hysteria over mega-muffins bewildering. For centuries, the Western aesthetic preferred women with some meat on their bones, to use the vernacular. Scholars have noted that from about 1400 to the late seventeenth century, the ideal body type for women was the "reproductive figure," which we might regard as attractively plenteous but C. Everett Koop would vilify as "fat." (One imagines Koop striding disgustedly through an exhibit of the religious art of the Middle Ages, harrumphing his displeasure at all those porcine cherubs and chunky angels and corpulent Madonnas.) By 1700, the feminine desideratum was full-figured, generously proportioned around bosom and bottom, but somewhat slenderer at the waist. Nevertheless, this "maternal" outline was "at least plump by any standard."[15]

By the 1920s, the rounded, the ample, the Rubenesque womanly shape was falling into fashionable disfavor; a smaller body, "with no remnant of the promising, reproductive tummy"[16] was in vogue. (And, soon, in *Vogue*.) Scholars call this type the sexual "free agent," built more for love-making than baby-making. She was lean; for the first time since the invention of movable type, thin was in—despite the lingering association in the popular mind between thinness and such ravaging diseases as tuberculosis.

Nags, who are always with us—it is only the object of the henpecking that changes—began hectoring American women to shed pounds, not so much as to attain comeliness as for a variety of sometimes dubious health-related reasons. Nor were men spared. Sarah Tyson Rorer, author of an astounding fifty-four cookbooks in the early years of the twentieth century, lectured, "Dainty cooking, not such as tempt men to gluttony, is what our housewives should study."[17] Again, the imagery is religious: men are tempted by the sin of overeating; gluttony, after all, is among the seven deadly sins.

Mrs. Rorer was "not slim,"[18] as Hillel Schwartz graciously notes in *Never Satisfied*, his cultural history of fat. Like her spiritual heir Dr. Koop—indeed, Mrs. Rorer was a Spiritualist, so we cannot discount the possibility that the Shape Up, America! commissars are channeling her at this very moment—Mrs. Rorer did not let the lard on her own belly keep her from pointing out the cellulite on her neighbor's thighs. (The exact details of Mrs. Rorer's hypocrisy are harder to document than those of Dr. Koop, who, as George Will recalled, showed up for a lunch with Will and Meg Greenfield and "washed down a cheeseburger and fries with two martinis."[19])

"An excess of flesh," Mrs. Rorer sniffed, "is to be looked upon as one of the most objectionable forms of disease, and must be treated as such."[20] Decades before Koop, she had hit on the disease angle: "The disease of obesity—for it certainly is a disease—creeps on so slowly that the individual becomes thoroughly wedded to the form of life producing it before he realizes his true condition." The answer: renounce fat, abjure sweets and sugar, at all costs do not touch the demon liquor or such devilish foods as potatoes, rice, or bread—staples of a healthy diet today. (Lest we snicker too long at the marks who bought Mrs. Rorer's books, a ridiculous book proclaiming that "refined sugar is lethal when ingested by humans"[21] sold more than a million copies in 1975. If a sucker was born every minute then, at least two seem to be born every minute today.)

The First World War broke out, and the diet zealots hitched their wagon to the caissons that went rolling along. The doughboy at the front had no more ferocious enemy than those on the home front whose shape resembled the Pillsbury doughboy. "Any healthy, normal individual, who is now getting fat is unpatriotic," shrieked Dr. Luella E. Axtell in 1919. (Dr. Axtell, who was 5 foot, 2 and 1/2 inches tall, had once assaulted the scales with 203 pounds, proving once again that no one sings louder in the church choir than the reformed whore.) Fat, as Hillel Schwartz writes, was now deemed "messy, dirty, poisonous." One 1918 medicine ad announced, "Auto-Intoxication [overeating, that is] More Deadly Than Warfare,"[22] which might be news to the soldiers who fought at Belleau Wood.

Nevertheless, doctors viewed the weight-loss game with a jaundiced eye. In 1926 Dr. Woods Hutchinson, former president of the American Medical Association, decried "this present onslaught upon one of the most peaceable, useful, and law-abiding of our tissues"—the dreaded FAT. In 1930, Dr. L.F. Barker of Johns Hopkins University mentioned that "the deliberate underfeeding by young girls and young women . . . is becoming a menace not only to the present, but to future generations."[24]

No research more vividly, even chillingly, illustrated the perils of excessive dieting than the work of Ancel Keys, whose Minnesota Experiment of 1944–1945 is written up in his massive 1,385 page, two-volume *The Biology of Human Starvation* (1950).

Keys' subjects were thirty-six conscientious objectors, most of them Quakers or members of the Church of the Brethren, who volunteered for a one-year study on the effects of semistarvation. Now, by "semistarvation" Keys did not mean a dollop of gruel and a strip of old shoe leather once a week. Rather, his subjects, after a three-month control period, went on a six-month 1,570-calorie-a-day diet, under which they were to lose from 19 to 28 percent of their body weight. (Regular exercise—three-mile-a-day walks and the performance of maintenance chores—helped keep them trim as well.) This was, as Dr. William Bennett and Joel Gurin noted in *The Dieter's Dilemma*, "the most detailed study of experimental starvation ever conducted on human beings."[25]

The six-month diet consisted primarily of whole-wheat bread, potatoes, turnips, cabbage, and grains: not the tastiest foods in the culinary world, but better than a Slim-Fast shake. And note that 1,570 calories a day actually *exceeds* the caloric limit of most current-day diets, which can be as low as an inhuman 600 calories a day.

So what happened to these thirty-six precocious weight-watchers? They lost weight, of course: an average of 24 percent of body weight and 50 percent of body fat. But before the Minnesota Cabbage and Turnip Diet becomes the next craze among would-be Kate Mosses, consider: The average heart volume of the subjects decreased by 20 percent. Average pulse rate plummeted from 56 to 37.8 beats a minute. Leg, back, and forearm strength decreased by an average of 30 percent. Testes size decreased. Men became moody (no wonder!), apathetic, and lethargic. They had blackouts, giddiness, and more combined neuroses than the cast of *Seinfeld*. They bit their nails; they quarreled; they paced restlessly. Two suffered nervous breakdowns. One chopped off a fingertip, apparently in a bid to rejoin the world of hamburger-eaters. They lost all interest in matters sexual and instead became obsessed with food. The less they ate, the more it consumed their thoughts. They became . . . well, bores. Their "mental activities narrowed to thinking about food."[26] The centerpiece, the cynosure, of their everyday lives was mealtime. Anyone who has lived with a fad dieter knows the story.

Gradually, they resumed regular eating. Yet "they remained miserable."[27] The menu became regular but the men did not. They became ravenous, gluttonous pigs. They ate, on average, more than 5,000 calories a day but still complained of hunger. They were insatiable, some of them eating three lunches—three *lunches*—a day.

Eventually, their weights returned to "normal." but it would be an additional nine months before the muscle they had lost would reappear. The experiment—the 1,570-calorie-a-day diet—had led to sickness, extreme weakness, even madness. Who could have known that within two to three decades, the Minnesota regimen would be par for the course for millions of desperate dieters?

The Minnesota Diet turned thirty-six healthy and enthusiastic volunteers into cranky, sickly, maladjusted sluggards. By any conceivable measure, these men were less happy when dieting (or rebounding) than they had been before. But Americans demand happiness—its pursuit, after all, is engraved in our Declaration of Independence—so the food-fighters sought to convince their countrymen that the old stereotype of the cheerful fat man was rubbish. No one with a wattle, a collop, a dewlap of flab could possibly be happy. A typical Metropolitan Life Insurance Company advertisement of 1941 showed Old King Cole, bulbous, contentedly smoking his pipe, attended by his fiddlers three, while the caption read, "We Hate To Disagree With Mother Goose."[28] But . . . no man could be a merry old soul with *that* caloric intake. (As for the pipe, we expect it would be airbrushed out of any ad today. Hadn't the old fool read the Surgeon General's report?)

"[O]ne cannot be too thin,"[29] declares an author of a recent book purporting to combat our "health crisis" of overweight Americans. The Minnesota starvelings might take issue with this, but if Jack Sprat, who could eat no fat, is a hero for our age, his wife, who could eat no lean, is a villainness. Or perhaps just a victim of the oppressive patriarchy. Poor Mrs. Sprat never met Susie Orbach, oracle of psychobabble and author of *Fat Is a Feminist Issue*.

"Fat," wrote Ms. Orbach, fatuously, "is a social disease, and fat is a feminist issue. Fat is not about lack of self-control or lack of willpower. Fat is about protection, sex, nurturance, strength, boundaries, mothering, substance, assertion, and rage. It is a response to the inequality of the sexes."[30]

And you thought you ate ice cream because you liked it.

Ms. Orbach went on to try out her theories on such clients as Princess Diana, who reacted to the inequality of the sexes embodied in flab by becoming the world's best-known bulimic, vomiting the food she ate, purging herself of "boundaries, mothering, substance" by disgorging her meals. This was sick and pathetic; Diana's aversion to fat helped make her a deeply unhappy person—but hey, she looked nice in a gown. And isn't that what *really* matters?

(If it's any consolation to Ms. Orbach, women constitute 90 percent of the clientele of commercial weight-loss clinics. And they make up almost all of the bulimics and anorexics in this thin-obsessed land.)

Today, you can't visit a bookstore without tripping over a rack of diet books. *Publishers Weekly*, the book review magazine, receives about thirty new diet and weight-loss titles every week.

The first nationwide weight-loss best-seller was Dr. Lulu Hunt Peters's 1917 tome *Diet and Health, with Key to the Calories*. Caloric intake played the starring role in the early years of the industry. "If you want to reduce, you must count calories,"[31] lectured a magazine in 1923. But the authors of these books eventually learned that while a sucker may be born every minute, a sucker is not willing to buy the same book over and over. So by 1961, a Rumanian-born obstetrician named Dr. Herman Taller was all the rage among the slim-obsessed with his book *Calories Don't Count*. Of course they do, but that didn't stop the book from clinging to the best-seller lists for almost a year. Serious nutritionists and physicians were aghast; it was "trash," fumed Frederick Stare of Harvard, who said, "There is hardly a word of sense in the whole book." Philip L. White of the American Medical Association's Council on Foods and Nutrition declared, "This book is a grave injustice to the intelligent public and can only result in considerable damage to the prestige of the medical profession."[32] If it was an insult, gullible Americans were eager to pay for the privilege: two million copies of *Calories Don't Count* were sold—until Dr. Taller exited Celebrity Nation after being convicted of various crimes, including mail fraud and conspiracy.

Fad diets went hand in hand with wonder pills in the mitts of the gullible. In the 1990s, women killed themselves with fen-phen, vouched for by none other than America's family doctor; in the 1930s, the killer miracle pill of choice was dinitrophenol, plumped for by none other than the *New Republic*, which would later act as a virtual press agent for Chick Koop, lauding his every banality as the wisdom of a rare sage.

Dinitrophenol, a derivative of benzene, was the fen-phen of its day. It had been used as an industrial toxin since the nineteenth century and was a critical ingredient in various explosive devices during the First World War: what better substance to slay that old demon, fat?

To women who wanted to trade in their rounded maternal forms for the newly fashionable litheness—"Why oh why couldn't I have been born in the fifteenth century?" one imagines the plangent chorus singing—dinitrophenol was greeted as a virtual savior. For this was no placebo, no worthless vial of Dr. Feelgood's Pounds-Off elixir. Dinitrophenol worked. By accelerating the dieter's metabolism, it made weight loss of two to three pounds a week almost a sure thing. By 1936, 100,000 people were popping this pill.

The only problem was, well, that it was an industrial toxin. In the words of Hillel Schwartz, "Dieters taking dinitrophenol felt warm."[33] (That was the least of their problems.) "They perspired. They noticed rashes forming on their skin. Some lost their sense of taste. Some went blind from cataracts. A few died. Whether they had bought Corpulean, Formula 37, or Slim, they were taking poison."

The fad passed. So too, alas, did some of the faddists.

The history of the diet biz is replete with scoundrels and mountebanks and hypocrites of Koopian proportions. There was Susan Powter, the screaming Amazonian author of *Stop the Insanity*! who, alas, seems not to have taken her own advice. Powter is to fat as C. Everett Koop is to tobacco, prompting Dr. Tom Sanders of Kings College, London to remark, "This obsession with eradicating fat entirely from our diet is no more than modern voodoo."[34]

Or take Dr. Stuart Berger, author of the best-selling trio *The Southampton Diet*, *Forever Young: Twenty Years Younger in Twenty Weeks*, and *The Immune Power Diet*. Berger was his own best advertisement, at least for a short while. An imposing 6'7", he had tipped—or should we say collapsed—the scales at 420 pounds before plummeting to a too-thin 208 pounds. He explained obesity as the product of food allergies—which was welcome news to the 98 percent of American adults who have no such allergies and can, presumably, gorge to their heart's content. Author Michael Fumento adds the coda to Berger's strange career:

> Unbeknownst to his clients and readers, Berger was a total glutton. Zabar's, his favorite New York delicatessen, shipped over a daily order of quail's eggs, sides of smoked salmon, several buckets of cream cheese and pickled herring, and dozens of bagels and roasted chickens. But while he fooled millions of Americans, there was somebody he couldn't deceive: that fellow who wears a hooded black robe and carries a scythe. In 1994 Berger died at age forty of a heart attack; he weighed 365 pounds.[35]

We have remarked upon Dr. Koop's curious fusion of religious and militaristic imagery. His faux-prophetic thunderings are not out of the mainstream of diet quackery; indeed, the 1970s saw a burst of absurd religio-dietary books that might have issued from Koop's pen, at least after his second martini of the day. As catalogued in Roberta Pollack Seid's *Never Too Thin: Why Women Are at War with Their Bodies*, there was *God's Answer to Fat—Lose It!* (1976) by Frances Hunter, the cheerfully titled *More of Jesus and Less of Me* (1976) by Joan

Cavanaugh, and *Help Lord—The Devil Wants Me Fat*! (1978)[36], in which author C.S. Lovett finds the Prince of Darkness himself in every Ho-Ho, Ding-Dong, and Dorito in the land. For tubbies of a prayerful bent, the Reverend H. Victor Kane even composed *Devotions of Dieters*, which featured such pre-meal offerings of grace as:

I promise not to sit and stuff
But stop when I have had enough. Amen.[37]

It is all very easy for us to snicker at charlatans who see the devil in fat, but what, if not the devil, does Dr. Koop see in cigarettes? (Perhaps these believers in a Slim-Fast Christ forgot their Luke 12:22: "And he said to his disciples, 'Therefore I tell you, do not be anxious about your lief, what you shall eat, nor about your body. . . . '")

Quacks believe that there is strength in numbers and that respectability can be purchased with a three-dollar word and an impressive letterhead. The nation's weight-loss doctors have always operated on the very margins of respectability, falling somewhere between faith healers and the lady who answers the phone at 3:00 A.M. when you call the Psychic Hotline. They needed an organization, an acronym, and they got one: the American Society of Bariatric Physicians, or the unpronounceable ASBP.

Bariatric is derived from the Greek word *baros*, or weight. So is ASBP in the Hippocratic tradition of Greek medicine? To use a Greek phrase, οῦ μῆ ("by no means"). George Blackburn of Harvard, a physician who treats obesity, has said, "You hear more weird endocrine, metabolic, nutritional gimmicks and beliefs if you talk informally to nine-tenths of the people in that society—they're as close to witchcraft as you can get." (According to two authors who braved an ASBP convention, "many of the bariatricians show a middle-age paunch; several are quite stout, and a few are frankly obese."[38] Witchdoctor, heal thyself!) The organization "has second-class professional standing,"[39] which is a polite way of saying that few of the top medical students are torn between becoming a brain surgeon and joining the wonderful world of bariatrics. Yet bariatric surgery "is one of the fastest growing specializations in the United States."[40]

The quest for respectability is one reason diet docs—excuse us, bariatricians—are so keen on classifying obesity as a "disease."

They can be fervent on the subject. "It was like a religious conversion," Dr. Jerry Darm, director of Weight Control Services at Providence Milwaukie Hospital in—no, neither Providence or Milwaukee—Portland, Oregon told science journalist Michael Fumento: "I suddenly realized that hypertension, heart disease, and diabetes are symptoms of the disease. The disease is obesity."[41] Unfortunately, like many conversion experiences, Dr. Darm's was intensely personal and not provable by scientific method.

But as millions of women starved themselves, popping pills and swilling inedible liquid concoctions, torturing themselves as images of Kate Moss and Cindy Crawford played in their mind's eyes, the sturdy outline of an uninvited truth began to take shape: diets don't work. The diet industry is a sham. And even in those rare cases in which pounds come off and stay off, the dieter is likely to wind up *less* healthy than before.

A 1992 National Institutes of Health study found that between 90 and 98 percent of dieters "regain the weight they lost, *plus* a little more, in the two years after they stop dieting"[42] (emphasis added). Or as one researcher has written, "If 'cure' from obesity is defined as reduction to ideal weight and maintenance of that weight for 5 years, a person is more likely to recover from most forms of cancer than from obesity."[43]

In one typical study of 121 "moderately obese" persons who lost over sixty pounds on supervised fasts, only 5.7 percent were able to maintain their reduced weights. Indeed, after nine years, 90 percent had reverted to their original weights.[44] Only the wallet is made lighter by the average diet.

A classic study in Denmark of fifty-seven overweight patients who were randomly assigned to either a very low calorie diet (VLCD) or horizontal gastroplasty surgery (popularly known as stomach stapling) found that both worked—at first, and for a very short time. The success rate (defined as keeping off at least half of their original loss) for the first year was 70 percent for the VLCD and 89 percent for surgery. And then the bottom fell out. Or should we say the bottom came back. By the end of year two, the success rate for the VLCD was just 38 percent; for surgery, it was 66 percent. By the end of year five, only 3 percent of those on the very low calorie diet and 16 percent of those who had gone under the surgeon's knife could be counted as "successes."[45]

The phenomenon of "yo-yo," or "cycling," dieting, is by now well-established in the literature of . . . dare we say . . . bariatrics. Loss, gain, loss, gain . . . the typical dieter is on a treadmill (perhaps Ferris wheel would be the more apposite image): she has the illusion of progress but she always ends up right back where she started. But not quite. For she is worse for the wear. As Dr. Wayne Calloway explains, "what you lose is not what you gain. You lose fat and muscle; you gain back primarily fat, and when you gain it back, it tends to come back in the belly, which is the area excess fat is most associated with complications such as heart attacks, diabetes, high blood pressure, and strokes."[46] The Framingham Heart Study, which we shall discuss later, found that persons with "high weight variability"—the yo-yoers—were from 25 to 100 percent likelier to suffer from heart disease or to die prematurely (strange phraseology; no doubt it will seem premature to each of us, even centenarians) than were those whose weight did not fluctuate. Dr. Glenn A. Gaesser, professor of exercise physiology at the University of Virginia and author of *Big Fat Lies*, notes, "Dieting almost always promotes the very thing it is supposed to cure, obesity."[47]

The complications from yo-yo dieting go far beyond the rebounding dieter being able to pinch an extra inch. Researchers who analyzed data from a 1957 Western Electric Study found that men "who gain and lose large amounts of weight in middle adulthood may have a 26 percent increased risk for death from coronary heart disease after age 40."[48]

Though Harvard men may frequently act as if the rules that the rest of us live by do not apply to them, even they cannot evade the grim logic of the yo-yo. Epidemiologist Steven N. Blair of the Cooper Institute for Aerobics Research in Dallas studied nonfatal disease in 12,205 male Harvard alums whose average age was 67. Almost a quarter (23.2 percent) of those who admitted to "always dieting" suffered from heart disease, more than double the number of those who "never" dieted (10.6 percent). The "always" dieters also suffered from higher rates of hypertension than the "never" dieting (38.3–23.4 percent) and a greater incidence of diabetes (14.6–3.0 percent). Among those who admitted to "sometimes" dieting, the more frequent the dieting, the higher the incidence of illness. All of which led Blair to conclude, "One of the fundamental tenets of the weight loss industry is if you get people to eat less, they'll lose weight. And if they lose weight, they'll be better off. And there is no evidence to support either one."[49]

(Now and then, a study may suggest that dieting works wonders. The results are so impressive that they could almost have been written by a weight-loss center's advertising firm. Well, for all practical purposes, they were. A great deal of dieting "research receives funding from commercial weight loss companies,"[50] writes Frances M. Berg of the *Healthy Weight Journal*, and this tends to add to the general confusion, frustration and complexity in the obesity field." Rent-a-scholars give a good study—if the price is right.)

These subsidized studies never bother itemizing the health problems associated with dieting. Dr. Janet Polivy of the University of Toronto has documented a long and grim list of maladies directly attributable to weight loss:

- gallstones
- cardiac disorders
- fainting, weakness, and fatigue
- slowed—or increased—heart rate, depending on the disorder
- elevated cholesterol
- anemia
- gouty arthritis
- edema
- headache
- nausea
- hair loss and thinning hair
- hypertension
- diarrhea and constipation
- aching muscles
- abdominal pain
- elevated uric acid levels
- cold intolerance
- loss of lean tissue
- changes in liver function
- dry skin
- muscle cramps
- amenorrhea and decreased libido
- refeeding complications from fasting diets, such as edema, potassium deficiencies, biliary tract disorders, pancreatic complications
- death.[51]

Very low calorie diets of less than 800 calories have been linked with "sudden and potentially fatal cardiac arrhythmias" by the Michigan Health Council. Dr. Nancy Wellman, President of the American Dietetic Association, has cautioned that "the most significant drawback to these diets is the potential for life-threatening side effects. . . . The loss of body protein—and here we are talking about muscle tissue—may affect cardiac function and could be related to heart failure."[52]

Admittedly, death is unlikely to visit most women slurping up their Whatever-Fast diet drinks, twirling a sprig of parsley around their bony fingers while dreaming of hot fudge sundaes and banana splits. But the nonfatal side effects of VLCDs are enough to drive a woman to Prozac. Anxiety, depression, emotional withdrawal, and a decreased attention span are common. So is halitosis, or as the Michigan Health Council undaintily put it, "strong, unpleasant breath and body odor."[53] Be thankful you've never gotten a whiff of Cindy Crawford.

Frances M. Berg of the *Healthy Weight Journal* has remarked on the tendency of women to take up vegetarianism in their flight from fat. Yet not "only is this a futile effort—research shows American women are more likely to get their fat from baked goods and desserts than from meat—but it can lead to nutrition deficiencies, fatigue, apathy and irritability."[54] A vegetarian diet invites anemia and listlessness—not exactly the New You you might be hoping for.

The unsavoriness of the typical diet may actually vitiate the nutritional value of the meal. Researchers have found that in subjects who anticipate a bland or lousy meal, the brain informs the stomach, which in turn may undersecrete the gastric juices that break down the food. Gastroenterologist Robert Russell, associate director of the USDA Human Nutrition Research Center at Tufts University, says, "If you really hate the food, or if you don't anticipate pleasure, your secretions will be less, and that could affect bioavailability"[55] of nutrients. So just *thinking* about that Jenny Craig patty sends your stomach a signal: Slow Down/Depressing Matter En Route.

* * *

Postwar America was nothing if not organization-mad, and those in search of slimness began joining groups. Take Off Pounds Sensibly (TOPS) took off in 1948. Overeaters Anonymous, patterned after Alcoholics Anonymous (devotees of rum cake might join both), started in 1960, and it was followed a year later by the heavyweight champion of dieting businesses, Weight Watchers.

Weight Watchers, which as we shall see has become a very generous sponsor of Dr. Koop, he who does so enjoy watching the weights of others, if not himself, was launched in the same year that two million Americans were learning that *Calories Don't Count* from the soon-to-be-felonious Dr. Herman Taller. Weight Watchers was not, however, born in mountebankery. It was, instead, hatched in the apartment of a 214–pound New York City woman named Jean Nidetch. She and six overweight friends gathered for moral support as they fought their battles of the bulge; Nidetch, at least, was successful, dropping seventy-two pounds. Her neighborly idea of friends helping friends diet was eventually swallowed by H.J. Heinz, which has turned Weight Watchers into a Heinz-enriching scheme that makes about two-thirds of its money from the Heinz products sold to clients.

From its beginnings as a kind of coffee-but-no-dessert klatch, Weight Watchers grew from $160,000 in revenues in 1964 to $8 million in 1970 to $39 million in 1977 to a hefty $1.35 billion in 1995. After ponying up a registration fee and weekly meeting payments for six weeks, the conscientious weight watcher—of whom there are upwards of half a million at any given time—will breakfast, lunch, and dine on the low-fat, low-taste cuisine bearing the distinctive Weight Watchers seal. Weight Watchers is more than a diet buddy: it's a lifestyle, or so its managers insist. Vice President of Marketing Len Tacconi says, "Weight Watchers members don't think of themselves as former customers. They think of themselves as being on a break."[56] Sort of like Scientology, apparently: in once, in for life.

The company's timing has not always been impeccable. With great hullabaloo and a contract worth $1 million annually, it signed up as a spokeswoman Sarah Ferguson, Princess Diana's floozy sister-in-law. The oft-maligned "Duchess of Pork," whose obsession with her waistline was almost as pathetic as that of the never-thin-enough Diana, signed a piece of direct mail that landed in the mailboxes of two million American dieters days before Diana's death in an automobile accident. Losing weight, joked Fergy, was "harder than outrunning the paparazzi." Oops! The admen worked overtime revamping the Duchess's print and TV commercials, making her somber, serious, and overflowing with "empathy with people afflicted by obesity and eating disorders."[57]

The Duchess was the first member, or at least ex-member, of the royal family to endorse a commercial product. Why Weight Watchers? Well, why not? She had never tried the program until shortly before she signed on the $1 million dotted line. She was then in the thin cycle of her yo-yoing weight, and this loss had occurred quite without the intervention of Heinz's finest. Thus, as Michael Lewis wrote in the *New York Times*, "Weight Watchers cannot honestly imply that it helped a Duchess to lose weight, though of course the company will."[58]

"If I can do it, anyone can," chirped the Duchess in her post-mourning TV commercials. (She was speaking of losing weight, not marrying a dimwitted prince and making off with a lucrative alimony settlement.) And the con worked. Weight Watchers' membership shot upward after some sluggish years.

The Duchess was an appropriate spokeswoman for Weight Watchers, which fancies itself the class act of the diet industry; indeed, at times it appears embarrassed by the company it keeps. (Then again, can you blame it? What self-respecting firm wouldn't be just a bit red-faced about sharing a market niche with the likes of Richard Simmons Slimmons, with its "Project Me" motivation tapes for only $25 a pop, its "Dance Your Pants Off" aerobics video, and, even more trepidation-inducing than a one-way ticket on the *Titanic*, a pass aboard the seafaring Richard Simmons Cruise to Lose?)

The haughtiness of Weight Watchers was evident in the testimony of Charles M. Berger, President of Weight Watchers International, before the May 7, 1990 hearings on "Deception and Fraud in the Diet Industry" conducted by the Subcommittee on Regulation, Business Opportunities, and Energy of the U.S. House of Representatives' Committee on Small Business.

The hearings were chaired by a publicity-mad nonentity named Ron Wyden (D-OR), who went on to become a publicity-mad nonentity in the Senate. Nevertheless, they did throw a sometimes sharply illuminating light on the perils and false promises of pills and fad diets.

Mr. Berger was the lead witness, befitting his company's leading role in the industry, and his was the sort of smarmy, sanctimonious performance that gives suck-ups a bad name. Playing to the Democrat Wyden's partisan instincts, Berger primly noted that *certain* "companies in our field"—far be it from him to name names, wink wink—had adopted the "extreme" methods of 1980s Wall Street. The decade of greed! With model tartuffery, Berger stated, "public health is a very important matter for the United States, and it can't be left to industry self-policing."[59] In other words, bring on the regulators! (As volume upon volume of economic history has shown, regulatory agencies usually become captive of the largest and most influential big businesses—the ones, say, that can buy a piece of someone like C. Everett Koop. They use that influence to write regulations that punish their competitors. Not that Weight Watchers would ever *dream* of doing such a thing.)

As Mr. Berger told the subcommittee:

> I will say that we honestly do believe that this is an instance where Government and congressional regulation would work better, and I would like to cite for example, if you will permit me, the fact that our parent company, the H.J. Heinz Co., founder, Henry J. Heinz, was instrumental in the passage of the first food and drug laws in 1906, much to the consternation of many of his competitors and colleagues in the food industry. We feel the same way today.[60]

And so Mr. Berger left the witness table, the consummate brownnose having just stroked the teacher, and it is not so hard to imagine him sticking out his tongue at his competitors, giving them a snotty chorus of "nyah-nyah-nyah-nyah-nyah."

"[W]e do appreciate your call for additional regulation,"[61] Congressman Wyden saluted him.

The remaining executives came on to do their own apple-polishing, though none were so oleaginously successful as Mr. Berger. The second-largest diet program, Jenny Craig, whose annual revenues are the in range of $400 million and whose American clientele at any given time numbers about 90,000, was founded in 1983 by husband and wife Sid and Jenny Craig. After a substantial enrollment fee, the dieter must purchase from the diet centers barely edible Jenny Craig meals, ostensibly such dishes as Fish Festiva and Pasta Primavera, which can run close to $100 a week. The corpulent comedienne Beth Donahue jokes, "Jenny's ads say you can 'Sign up now for just six cents a pound.' What they don't tell you is that you should cash in all your 401K savings if you want to be able to afford Jenny's 'cuisine.'"[62] (Jenny Craig makes almost all its profits from the sales of its food; Weight Watchers makes about two-thirds of its profits from its Heinz victuals.)

At the time of the Wyden hearing, Jenny Craig was flying high. Sid Craig, a former ballroom dance teacher who as a boy had tap-danced in the *Our Gang* comedies—not the sort of behavior likely to charm the hellion hearts of Spanky and Alfalfa—spoke publicly of annual revenue growth of 15 to 20 percent as far as the eye could see. Sid does not lack for self-confidence. "I always knew I'd own a limousine someday," he told *Forbes*. He met the charming Jenny, soon to be namesake of her very own New York Stock Exchange company, when he owned and she worked at a New Orleans diet center named Body Contour. Soon, as *Forbes* delicately put it, "they were divorced from their respective spouses"[63] and married each other. They sold Body Contour to rival Nutri/System in 1982, and decamped to Australia, where they founded the Jenny Craig centers. After a two-year "noncompete agreement" with Nutri/System expired, Jenny Craig invaded the United States and soon left Nutri/System eating its dust. (Which may well have tasted better than the typical Jenny Craig cuisine.)

Jenny Craig grew like a client on a fried chicken and milkshake diet. It added 100 centers a year through the early 1990s, and the ever-optimistic Sid Craig bragged, "We plan on blanketing the entire North American continent."[64] Given that the average Jenny Craig client stayed on the program for four months, Sid's grandiose vision must have included dragging into Jenny Craig centers, by hook or crook, every last American, even those who are already thin.

Jenny Craig's Vice President for Operations, Ellen Destray, also pronounced herself "pleased" to be hailed before Congressman Wyden's inquisition. She assured the solons that Jenny Craig was not a "quick-fix or a very low calorie diet."[65] No sirree: women on the Jenny Craig plan can wolf down a whole 1,000 calories a day, while men pig out on between 1,200 and 1,400 calories each day—or from 10 to 20 percent *fewer* calories than the subjects in the Minnesota starvation diet were fed. So if you should see on the street a flock of nervous, irritable, impotent men who talk of nothing but food, odds are there's a Jenny Craig near you. (The other weight-loss programs also fall below the Minnesota threshold. The typical Weight Watchers client consumes 1,250–1,500 calories a day, a Nutri/System client gets 1,200 calories a day, Optifast permits its dupes 800–1,200 calories a day, and Medifast starves its patients on from 500–1,500 calories a day.)

At the Wyden hearing, all of the CEOs and vice presidents of this or that hastened to point out that theirs was a scrupulously scientific regimen, leagues removed from the "many fad or quack diets . . . which are dangerous and at best useless,"[66] in the somber words of Charles E. Sekeres, President and CEO of Physicians Weight Loss Centers of America, Inc. After all, as Allan N. Stewart, President and CEO of Diet Center, Inc., said, "There are no quick fixes . . . no effortless miracle cures."[67] (Fen-phen would be sold as such in a couple of years, but we're getting ahead of ourselves.)

The usually meager qualifications of the "counselors" who staff these organizations came in for especial condemnation—"millions of Americans are participating in rapid weight-loss programs supervised by people . . . with little or no knowledge, training, or understanding of the complications of semistarvation,"[68] said Dr. Wayne Calloway, professor of medicine at George Washington University and the former vice president of the American Board of Nutrition. But an emphasis on credentialism misses the point, to wit, that this whole industry is a sham, and that diet doctors with parchment on the wall are even bigger shammers than a Jenny Craig counselor, and that, increasingly, it is the U.S. government, with its draconian body-weight charts and national nannyism, that is fueling this mad rush to semistarvation.

The Wyden hearings—there were three in 1990 and one in 1992—had their share of the inevitable, and apparently unintended, puns. "There is no question that childhood obesity is growing,"[69] declared the chairman, and who could disagree?

But there were also poignant moments, particularly from the parents of girls who had died as a result of consuming the pills and diuretics and laxatives of the snake-oil salesmen. (Almost 7 percent of American girls use diet pills.) Mr. and Mrs. Anthony Smith of State Center, Iowa—quintessential Middle Americans, even in geography—told of losing their pretty 20-year-old daughter Noelle: "Noelle died when her heart stopped as a result of an electrolyte imbalance that occurs when the body's potassium levels are so depleted as to cause an irregular heartbeat. Her potassium level was depleted as a result of the diet pills and diet regimes that she followed in her ceaseless efforts to lose weight."[70]

The subcommittee also heard from Dr. David F. Williamson, an epidemiologist in the Division of Nutrition of the Centers for Disease Control. Dr. Williamson, after repeating what is common knowledge everywhere outside a Weight Watchers program—"that the vast majority of obese persons are not successful in maintaining their initial weight loss longer than one year"—went on to warn that "[r]epeated dieting may be hazardous to one's health . . . there is increasing evidence that repeated cycles of weight loss, followed by weight gain, may have deleterious effects on health."[71]

This information was too late for Noelle Smith. And despite her parents' wishes, the drumbeat for weight loss goes on, and no one beats the skins with as much gusto as America's family doctor.

* * *

The diet industry underwent a most unwelcome slimming down of its own in the early 1990s. Its heftiest companies—Jenny Craig, Nutri/System Inc. (which made enough money to allow founder Harold Katz to buy the Philadelphia 76ers basketball team), and Weight Watchers—were "losing business rapidly."[72] Well over 1,000 diet centers closed within a couple of years. Weight Watchers virtually collapsed, shedding employees like easy-to-lose pounds and going from a $45 million profit in 1992 to a loss of $50 million two years later. Its Heinz-manufactured frozen foods were being challenged at the cash register by Nestlè's Lean Cuisine and ConAgra Inc.'s Healthy Choice. As late as 1997 Heinz closed fifty-five of its Weight Watchers centers; there was even speculation that Heinz might sell off the company. Jenny Craig, which operated 820 weight-management centers in the United States, saw its earnings plummet 84 percent in its second quarter of fiscal 1993 and sag for the remainder of the decade. Earnings per share in 1994 were "anorexic,"[73] according to the *San Diego Union-Tribune*. The initial membership fee was cut from $185 to $49, to no avail. A high-profile sex-discrimination lawsuit by eight male employees of Jenny Craig's Boston office drew a national chorus of guffaws directed at the organization. (It seems that the women asked this sad sack octet to shovel snow in the winter and subjected them to ceaseless chatter about "who to marry, who is pregnant, how to get pregnant."[74] One might think that the avoirdupois associated with childbearing defeats the whole Jenny Craig purpose, but there are higher callings in life than weight loss, after all.)

In 1993, the FTC initiated a deceptive-advertising claim against Jenny Craig that would drag on for four years before a settlement that required the company to inject just a wee bit of honesty into its ads, which are notable for their before and after shots of blowzy, obese women miraculously made svelte on just a few dollars a day. A similar complaint lodged against Weight Watchers resulted in the company's painful admission that "for many dieters weight loss is temporary."[75] Which ought to raise the question among potential clients: Unless my aim is temporary weight loss—say, to fit into a prom or wedding dress—why bother? Weight Watchers was also taken to task for boasting that it was superior to these other fly-by-night operations—a piece of braggadocio for which it had not a shred of evidence.

Also in 1993, Nutri/System declared bankruptcy and closed more than 300 of its centers. Panic set in. Which was an amusing irony: an industry that had fattened on the panic of others was now in full-scale panic itself. Nutri-System, Jenny Craig, and Diet Center began peddling fen-phen—which operated something like a diet in reverse: the companies fattened on it at first, then lost their shirts, if not their bellies. (As usual, bad, albeit unintentional, puns abounded. "Weight Watchers is not a growth business,"[76] remarked analyst Terry Bivens of Argus Research in New York. "Heinz Plan Trims Weight Watchers,"[77] yuk-yukked *USA Today*. *Newsday* headlined, "Weight Watchers Feels Corporate Belt-Tightening."[78] *Business Week* jested that "the diet market is starting to suffer from indigestion."[79] All of which is to say that the authors are not alone in committing the occasional offense against good taste and high-brow humor.)

Diet drinks, the best known being Slim*Fast, enjoyed a brief vogue in the late 1980s, until, as Michael Fumento has pointed out, the highly visible spokesmen (Los Angeles Dodgers' manager Tommy Lasorda, NBC weatherman Willard Scott) "became fat again."[80] Whereupon "Ultra Slim*Fast" came into being. These shakes are intended to replace one or two meals a day: they provide calcium, protein, fiber, and a gnawing hunger in your stomach and pain in your head. What a deal! True, Optifast helped Oprah Winfrey shed sixty-seven pounds in 1987—but those pounds came back with a vengeance.

The marketers of three liquid diets—Ultrafast, Medifast, and Optifast—Fast! Fast! Get it?—were cited by the Federal Trade Commission for such "deceptive and unsubstantiated advertising claims"[81] as Optifast's motto, "The One That's Clinically Proven Safe and Effective." These liquid diets, which are barely more nutritionally satisfying than the Chinese water torture, usually mandate an intake of from 420 to 800 calories a day for twelve to sixteen weeks—that is, starvation for three to four months—followed by a refeeding period that boosts the dieter to a still unreasonably low 1,000–1,200 calories a day. So that's all there is to it: choke down shakes that taste like motor oil for a few months, then nibble on Ally McBeal food for the rest of your life and you, too, can achieve a figure to die for. No wonder Tommy Lasorda would rather be fat. (The Medifast diet is just 450–500 calories a day: an intake so low the Geneva Convention probably outlaws it for prisoners of war.)

For a discouraging number of young women, the alternative to unsavory shakes is anorexia or bulimia. One in 500 American girls is starving herself through anorexia nervosa; perhaps one in fifty alternates binge eating with vomiting, the m.o. of the bulimic. Often, dieting is the critical link between a girl's dissatisfaction with her weight and her descent into the nightmares of starvation or binge and purge. "Eating disorders should be called 'dieting disorders,' because it is the dieting process and not eating that causes the initiation of both anorexia nervosa and bulimia nervosa,"[82] argues eating disorder specialist Joe McVoy of Springwood Hospital in Leesburg, Virginia.

The bottom fell out of the industry—briefly, at least. Weight Watchers has since rebounded, while Jenny Craig has not—for a variety of reasons, some good and others not-so-good. Heinz, grasping for alibis, blamed everything from the Lillehammer Olympics to the Los Angeles earthquake to cold winters. Mother Nature's fault, it seems. Less frantic observers noted that various appetite suppressants and "meal replacements" were gobbling up market share: some dieters were changing tactics, switching to Thompson Medical Inc.'s Slim-Fast powder and Dexatrim pills. Others, perhaps feeling the pocketbook pinch of expensive diet centers, were opting for cheaper health clubs. And as Jenny Craig officials admitted, "the extensive publicity that accompanied the introduction of Redux heightened the public's interest in weight loss pharmaceuticals, and appears to be responsible for softened demand being experienced by the Company for its products and services."[83] Jenny Craig "leads" slumped some 33 percent in the summer of 1996, as Redux took the field. (Not that Jenny Craig was pure of heart in the matter: it, unlike Weight Watchers, peddled Redux.)

Some Americans stopped looking to Jenny Craig to save their lives and started looking at the man or woman in the mirror. The astute few were realizing that pounds that came off did not stay off: "We're losing the war [on fat] as the industry is booming,"[84] said the director of the Nutrition Research Clinic of the Baylor College of Medicine. (Also booming was that segment of the fashion industry that caters to overweight women: in 1997, it sold more than $23 billion in women's apparel—or one quarter of all apparel sales—in size 16 or larger. This was an increase of 15 percent over two years.)

And last, but certainly not least, "a nascent anti-diet movement"[85] was "gaining a foothold."

Provocative books challenging the thinness-at-all-costs ethic—Laura Fraser's *Losing It: False Hopes and Fat Profits in the Diet Industry* and Dr. Glenn Gaesser's *Big Fat Lies*, to cite two examples—started showing up on bookshelves previously dominated by the Chicken Littles of the little-is-better school. A *Newsweek* cover story, relying heavily on Fraser, asked, "Is Fat That Bad?" and even to ask the question was a breakthrough.

The anti-dieting movement was not just another outgrowth in the garden of self-esteem; it was based on more than the need for tubbies to accept their own ampleness. It drew upon solid evidence; unlike the frantic claims of the diet industry, it had science on its side.

The tide began to turn in the 1980s. Study after study of group upon group found that, as Robert Pollack Seid writes, "Whether evaluating scale weight or lean-to-fat ratios—and even when people who were thinner because of smoking, cancer, or some pre-existing condition were carefully screened . . . [n]one of them showed that thinner was healthier."[86]

Indeed, quite the opposite. Take the legendary Framingham, Massachusetts cardiovascular study, in which 5,209 men and women were examined at intervals for thirty years. This was an enormous sample: about half the town's population between the ages of thirty and fifty-nine participated in an effort to better understand the causes of heart disease and strokes. When year thirty rolled around, the researchers were astounded by the results: the thinnest men were the deadest men.

Dr. Ancel Keys, he of the Minnesota starvation experiment, evaluated subjects in countries including Japan, Greece, Italy, Yugoslavia, Holland, Finland, and the United States. His conclusion, after decades of research: "The idea has been greatly oversold that the risk of dying prematurely or of having a heart attack is directly related to relative body weight. For middle-aged men, the best prospect for avoiding death in ten or fifteen years is to be about average, or a bit over, in relative weight."[87] Something like, say, C. Everett Koop's 6'1", 210 pounds. The sort of body one achieves after years of diligent red-meat eating, martini-drinking, and macadamia-nut-popping.

In a survey of almost a dozen population studies from Europe and the United States, Dr. Reubin Andres, clinical director of the National Institute on Aging, found that those who gain a modest amount of weight—another chin, a small spare tire, a pinchable inch or two—have the *lowest* mortality rates. "There's every reason to expect that truly obese people would benefit from losing weight," Andres told *Newsweek* in its pathbreaking cover story, "but if you look at survival, not at individual risk factors, those that lose do badly. We don't understand why."[88] What they do understand is that exercise, not diet, is the key to fitness, and by exercise they do not mean three hours pumping iron followed by an hour on the track. A nice daily walk will do just fine, thank you. But then again one does not need the ministrations and exhortations of Dr. Koop and the nags in order to walk—and scarce indeed is the federal agency or commercial weight-loss program that will subsidize a Koop Center for Brisk Walking.

A heavy person who is physically active is better off than a rail-thin person whose only exercise is flipping the remote control. Exercise is not an efficient way to lose weight; as *Big Fat Lies* author Glenn A. Gaesser says, "I never pitch exercise as means to lose weight, because most people will not lose a lot of weight."[89] One can be fat and fit; it is far more difficult to be fat, fit, and sedentary. "The distribution of fat within the body can be as important, or more so, than mere poundage: 'fat padding your waist and belly, giving you an apple shape . . . does the most damage to health. Fat hips and thighs, which give you that much-maligned pear shape, may injure only the ego."[90] Pear-shaped persons with substantial hips and thighs are at considerably lower risk of heart disease than are the apple-shaped. It's almost as difficult to change the fruits we resemble as it is to switch eye color: sucking down Slim*Fast shakes or nibbling at Jenny Craig's noodles sure aren't going to turn an apple into a pear.

Decades of weight and mortality studies have shown, according to Seid, that "Thinner was not better. Indeed, to the extent that there was a linear relationship between weight and mortality, it went in the *wrong* direction: Life expectancy was worst among the leanest in the populations, and in many instances best among the fattest."[91]

Good news for diet-breakers; not-so-good news for the diet police. But the news has not been widely disseminated. Certainly Dr. Koop was in no hurry to start spreading the news. In 1996 he told *Barron's*, "It doesn't often appear on the death certificate, but obesity is often the real cause of death."[92] Typically, Professor of Medicine JoAnn E. Manson of the Harvard Medical School wrote in 1997, "Overweight also contributes to . . . premature death"[93]—a wildly premature, or perhaps anachronistic, statement.

For it is just as possible, as Professor David M. Garner of the Michigan State University Department of Psychiatry told the Wyden subcommittee, that "the health risks associated with obesity (the primary rationalization for treatment) have been grossly exaggerated and, in fact, dieting (the supposed cure for obesity) may be more dangerous than obesity itself."[94] This is rank heresy in the kingdom of the thin. Garner compounded his sin by ridiculing the campaigns by the national nannies to get America to shape up. Observing that study after study shows that underweight persons are likelier to die young than are those of moderate or even heavy weights, he remarked, "To my knowledge, there have been no major health campaigns designed to encourage those below the national weight norms to embark on a program of weight gain in order to improve their health."[95] Bulk Up, America! The life you save may be your own.

A 1992 National Institutes of Health Technology Assessment Conference on Methods for Voluntary Weight Loss and Control was another turning point in the battle of the bulge-reducers. The NIH conference concluded that diet programs simply don't work: "Most people who achieve weight loss with any of these [commercial] methods regain weight."[96] Fasting and very low calorie diets were cited for a multitude of unpleasant effects, among them hair loss, dizziness, fatigue, and gallstones and acute gallbladder disease. These can be especially severe when relatively lean persons diet. According to Dr. Wayne Calloway, "within 8 weeks on a 520-calorie diet, as many as 25 percent of people will develop gallstones."[97] (What a bargain: lose a few pounds as well as your hair, your energy, your balance, and your gallbladder.)

Summing up the conference consensus, research physician Jules Hirsch of Rockefeller University in New York City stated,

> It is generally agreed that individuals who enter any of the available commercial programs may do so with high resolve and, therefore, lose weight in the short run. There is, however, a high dropout rate. No statistically sound evidence was presented at the conference to indicate that commercial, nonmedical programs have any enduring efficacy. When various programs with physician oversight and medical involvement were evaluated, it was found that approximately 50% of those who begin such programs drop out within the first year. Of those who remain, a third to one-half will lose a significant amount of weight and maintain a majority of the weight loss for a one-year period. Data for continued success beyond one year are very few. The consensus is that, by two years and surely by five years, the majority of subjects beginning any weight loss program will have returned to their starting weight. Probably fewer than 5% of those beginning the program will lose the weight and maintain it for as long as five years.[98]

(This information, too, has escaped the capacious ken of Dr. C. Everett Koop. In 1996 he went to bat for the diet industry, telling

Barron's, "It's not hard to lose weight but it is hard to keep the weight off. Weight Watchers and Jenny Craig both offer maintenance programs that can help on this score."[99] And they can help on other scores, as well, for both outfits pledged substantial sums to Shape Up America! and the personal fiefdom of Dr. Koop. The good doctor said upon leaving his surgeon general post that his integrity was not for sale, but then canny investors know that sometimes the real money can be made in frequent rentals.)

Critically, the NIH conferees emphasized the lack of evidence associating weight loss with reduced mortality. Indeed, just the opposite seems to be true. "Most epidemiologic studies suggest that weight loss is associated with increased mortality. . . ."[100]

Several speakers at the NIH conference reported on this surprising, yet consistent, evidence. Weight loss is associated with mortality, even when controlling for those who die of smoking-related diseases. After examining ten "widely varying studies," Dr. Reubin Andres of the NIH's National Institute on Aging Gerontology Research Center concluded, "For the general population, the results of the 10 studies do not support the idea that losing weight will increase longevity . . . [but] the opposite conclusion. If body weight for optimal survival increases with age, then weight gain with passage of time is permissible and can even be recommended."[101]

Which may explain why Dr. Koop, despite his fat subsidy from Weight Watchers, prefers to watch the weights of others, and why he is still going stout and strong in his eighties.

* * *

An editorial in the January 1, 1998 issue of the *New England Journal of Medicine* summarized the current state of knowledge on the link between obesity and illness. Drawing on the now-voluminous evidence on obesity, diet, and illness, the editorialists wrote, "Given the enormous social pressure to lose weight, one might suppose there is clear and overwhelming evidence of the risks of obesity and the benefits of weight loss. Unfortunately, data linking overweight and death, as well as the data showing the beneficial effects of weight loss, are limited, fragmentary, and often ambiguous."[102] (Much of this "ambiguous" evidence had appeared in several pathbreaking articles in the *NEJM* in the mid-1990s.)

The editorialists did much more than simply survey confusion. They charged that the up to $50 billion a year Americans spend on dieting and its various gimmicks "is wasted." The diet industry, they asserted, feeds on "guilt and self-hatred" which manifests itself in the anorexia and bulimia of young women. They even stuck up for the sensual—and soon to be sinful?—experience of gustatory pleasure. "Many Americans," they concluded, "are sacrificing their appreciation of one of the great pleasures of life—eating—in an attempt to look like our semi-starved celebrities."[103]

Now they had gone too far. This was heresy to the ideologists of Weight Loss Über Alles—the scolds of Shape Up or Ship Out, America—and heretics must be punished. Dr. Koop took the lead, for not only had the *NEJM* editorialists pooh-poohed his new hobbyhorse, they had even criticized the spectacle of "public health officials joining in the general enthusiasm for losing weight."[104] (Specifically Koop, according to footnotes.) So the Doctor attacked. He called the *New England Journal of Medicine* piece "a disappointing one that trivializes the second leading cause of preventable death in the United States."[105]

Denying that "the data linking overweight and death are limited, fragmentary, and often ambiguous," Koop and his sidekicks JoAnn Manson of Harvard Medical School and Theodore B. Van Itallie of Columbia University asserted, without evidence, that 20 percent of U.S. deaths from natural causes are due to "unhealthy weight." About 1.6 million Americans die of natural causes each year, so *voilà*!: 20 percent of 1.6 million is about 318,000. How dare the *New England Journal of Medicine* argue with *that* logic! For good measure, Koop and company affirmed that 318,000 was "a reasonable and conservative figure."[106] If you say so.

Yet, in responding, Koop unwittingly credited one of the editorialists' central points, which was that a major "reason for the medical campaign against obesity may have to do with a tendency to medicalize behavior we do not approve of."[107] Dr. Koop, for example, is offended by fat babies, lady smokers, pot-bellied men (himself excluded), and those who slather their hamburgers with melted Cheez-Whiz. But there remains enough of a libertarian streak in the American character that the medical meddler cannot simply point to the pot-bellied fellow and yell "Ban Him!" No, he must instead demonstrate that the pot-bellied man is in the grips of a disease, an illness—compulsive overeating, chocoholism—that so impairs his judgment that he is incapable of making the *right choice*. (As a prominent anti-tobacco crusader replied in 1997 to a question about individual choice, "People who are making decisions for themselves don't always come up with the right answer."[108]) This is why the stakes of the "debate" over whether or not obesity is a disease, as the Diet—or Else—partisans started arguing in the 1980s, are huge. Those stakes are not just, well, steaks, but freedom as well.

If obesity is a disease, if the Koops succeed in medicalizing avoirdupois, then the pot-bellied man must be forcibly slimmed—For His Own Good. This will be done with the usual mix of carrots and sticks, but since carrots are food—and food makes fat—the stick will become proportionally bigger over time. The things that make a man pot-bellied will be banned—or at the very least taxed to discourage consumption, with the revenues earmarked for Those Who Know Best so that they can "educate" the great unwashed—with as little political debate as possible, for after all this is a *medical* matter, and just as we don't entrust Joe Blow off the street with the responsibility to perform brain surgery, nor should we allow poor Joe the privilege of designing his own diet.

Jacob Sullum, in his book *For Your Own Good: The Anti-Smoking Crusade and the Tyranny of Public Health*, fancifully imagines a regulatory apparatus suitable for effective weight-loss: "In several states, people have to bring their cars to an approved garage for periodic emissions testing; there's no logistical reason why they could not also be required to weigh in at an approved doctor's office, say, once a year, reporting the results" to whatever government agency was in charge of Citizen Weight Loss. (Perhaps a newly empowered Bureau of Weights and Measures?) This plan is "ridiculous," writes Sullum, "because it's an odious intrusion by the state into matters that should remain private." At least it seems so today, although assistant secretary Philip R. Lee of the Department of Health and Human Services has whined that "The government is not doing enough" to combat obesity. "We don't have a coherent, across-the-board policy."[109] Mandatory weigh-ins, with appropriate punishments for the incorrigibly chunky (the force-feeding of lentils? Rosie O'Donnell photos plastered all over the refrigerator?), would at least be coherent and across-the-board, if coherently totalitarian and across-the-board tyrannical.

(Looking for an entertaining parlor game to play with refractory friends? How about a game of Design a Coherent Anti-Obesity Policy? The *Washington Times* has facetiously suggested a ban on "Happy

Meals"—how can fat children be happy, for goodness sake? And "high sales taxes on the likes of Oreo cookies to discourage consumption—but not too high lest the tax create a black market in Oreo cookies." And how about "a strict ban on sales of Ho-Hos and cupcakes to underage buyers," to be enforced by "random sting operations on convenience store owners."[110])

(Among the sweetest ironies of Koopian diet tyranny is that one of the most reliable methods of dieting is . . . to take up smoking. Puffing on the soon-to-be-forbidden weed alters the smoker's metabolism; it increases her "resting energy expenditure."[111] Swiss researchers discovered that smoking your way through twenty-four cigarettes a day boosts caloric expenditure by 10 percent; why use the Stair Master when a pack of Benson & Hedges will do just as well? Smokers understand this: surveys have shown that many young women smoke as a form of weight control. And it works the other way, too: "Quitting the habit causes weight gain in perhaps 80 percent of ex-smokers. Body weight increases on average from five to ten pounds."[112] A Brown University study of women on a very low calorie diet found that those who "successfully"[113] completed the program showed steadily increasing levels of codinine in the saliva, a tip off that their diets were complemented by greater consumption of the sinister weed.)

But back to the fat wars. The *New England Journal of Medicine* editors were seconded by the iconoclastic University of Virginia professor Glenn A. Gaesser, author of the myth-busting *Big Fat Lies*, who wrote the *NEJM* that "Health problems frequently blamed on excess body weight are more likely caused by an unhealthy lifestyle rather than obesity itself."[114]

As Dr. Garner of Michigan State told the congressional subcommittee, "Obesity is associated with a lowered incidence of certain cancers, respiratory disease, infectious disease, osteoporosis, and other ailments."[115] And belying Fatty Arbuckle's lament about the lovelessness of the obese, fat persons have a lower suicide rate than the thin. (Or perhaps nobody loves a fat man, but the thin may not even love themselves.)

Somewhat controversially, Garner and Dr. Susan Wooley of the University of Cincinnati Medical Center have argued that "It is difficult to find any scientific justification for the continued use of dietary treatments of obesity." They note that "[r]egardless of the specific techniques used, most participants regain the weight lost. There is remarkable consistency in the pattern of regain across behavioral, dietary and very low calorie diet approaches to obesity. Most approaches lead to weight loss during active treatment; however, most participants ultimately regain to levels that approximate their pre-treatment weight."[116]

"The great majority of people on weight-loss regimens are being treated, or are treating themselves, for a nondisease,"[117] state Dr. William Bennett and Joel Gurin. This is fighting Koop and his diet industry allies on the epidemiological high ground they have sought to occupy. The thinness police insist that the condition of overweightness is a "disease," and it is a disease very much like the common cold in that anyone can catch it. For instance, Harvard nutritionist Dr. Jean Mayer remarks ominously that "you can become very fat by eating just 1 percent more than you need every day."[118] *One* percent? If popping an extra cracker into your maw every night can make you "very fat," then who is safe? Never mentioned is the fact that there is less fat in the average American's diet today than in the past. "[O]ur diets are 33 to 34 percent fat now and they used to be 40 percent fat,"[119] according to epidemiologist Claude Bouchard. So from a fat-phobic's point of view, our diets are healthier today than ever before. But some facts are worthier of mention than others.

America's doctor, as we shall see in succeeding chapters, is a prime shill for weight loss. In so doing he is making America less healthy—not only physically but emotionally and mentally as well. As a former Jenny Craig counselor remembered one of her clients: "I was shocked. I looked at the client's chart before she started the program. She was five two and weighed 108 pounds. The computer said her weight range was 104 to 114, so they sold her a program to lose four pounds. Imagine! There is something wrong with that woman and it's not her weight."[120]

The woman is obviously a candidate for therapy, and not of the physical variety, but in a way she is only responding to the drumbeat of the diet crazies. The more we diet the fatter we get, and the cycle goes on and on until . . . well, as John Foreyt and Ken Goodrick put it in the *Lancet*, the medical journal, "Based on prevalence studies, from 1960 to 1991, we calculate that by the year 2230, 100% of adults in the USA will be overweight, as defined by a body mass index of more than 27."[121] (The body mass index nonsense is discussed in the next chapter.)

Foreyt and Goodrick were kidding—sort of. For no exaggeration is too preposterous for the diet hucksters. Which leads to the question: if obesity is a disease, is the obsession with obesity a disease of the mind? If Dom DeLuise is sick, is C. Everett Koop nuts?

3

Shape Up—Or Ship Out

"And ye shall eat the fat of the land."
—Genesis, XLV, 18

"Let me have men about me that are fat."
—*Julius Caesar*, Act I, Scene 2, Line 191

By the mid-1990s, the diet industry was in trouble. The "fat but fit" movement was gaining ground, if not weight. Thin-crazed dieters were gobbling fen-phen, not yet aware that it took pounds, and sometimes even years, off your life. Weight Watchers and its brethren were gasping and sputtering like a 300–pounder after a five-mile road race. Heinz was panicking: 13 percent of Heinz's sales worldwide come from Weight Watchers. As Jenny Craig officials admitted in the company's annual report to the Securities and Exchange Commission, "maintaining its market position and continued growth depend upon the Company's ability to attract new participants for the Program."[1] But it was no longer growing, and neither were its brethren in the field. And so to the rescue rode the knight in the white hat—or the Ruritanian Navy uniform—former Surgeon General C. Everett Koop.

It is said that when President Harry Truman asked Michigan Senator Arthur Vandenberg how he could get the American people behind his Cold War military buildup, Vandenberg replied, "Scare the hell out of them." Koop was not beneath doing that himself. For he minted one of those baseless statistical canards that become, through a process of repetition similar to that which enshrines such "urban legends" as alligators in the sewer and the "marriage" of Rock Hudson and Jim Nabors, widely accepted as fact. In December 1994, pontificating on the South Lawn of the White House, an adoring Hillary Clinton at his side ("I always do everything Dr. Koop tells me," she chirped), with the leading public health bureaucrats looking on and applauding dutifully, Dr. Koop launched Shape Up America! (SUA!), a "broad-based education initiative" to inform chronically clueless Americans about the benefits of "increased physical activity and healthy eating."[2] Exercise and eat right: if only we'd known!

Koop acted in an unusual partnership with the White House; as the *Washington Post* observed, "the newest recruit in the government's strategy to reduce fat is former U.S. surgeon general C. Everett Koop, drafted by the Clinton White House to help 'Shape Up America!'"[3] The military wannabe in Koop responded to this draft, if not to the one five decades ago: after all, this was deemed a "national mobilization," a locution to hasten the blood of any empire-builder. And from that very first day, Dr. Koop exhibited the same careful regard for truth that has distinguished the Clinton White House.

"After smoking, which causes an estimated 500,000 deaths annually, obesity-related conditions are the second leading cause of death in the U.S., resulting in about 300,000 lives lost each year,"[4] thundered the doctor with the certitude of the fanatic. For this claim was wholly bogus, spun almost out of thin air.

As a 1998 *Wall Street Journal* investigation found, Koop defended the "300,000 deaths" figure by pointing to a paper in the November 1993 issue of the *Journal of the American Medical Association*. There was only one small problem: the article "never said obesity killed that many people." It merely said that "dietary factors" and sedentary lifestyle may be responsible for 300,000 deaths a year. It did not call obesity "a disease"[5]: that bizarre interpretation was taken up by Dr. Koop and a gaggle of drug companies seeking FDA approval for Redux and other fat-fighting drugs.

Those doctors not on the payroll of pharmaceutical companies or the C. Everett Koop empire generally agree with Marcia Angell, who wrote in the *New England Journal of Medicine* that obesity is "no more of a disease than bank robbery is a disease."[6] But fortunes hung on this definition, and on Dr. Koop's magic number. "The 300,000 figure was the single most important reason the advisory committee approved Redux," said Lynn McAfee of the Council on Size and Weight Discrimination. "And it's a fake number."[7] (Among other things, it relies on the assumption that breast cancer is caused by fat—a fallacy convincingly refuted in 1999 by the Nurses Health Study, a fourteen-year tracking of 88,795 women which found no link between fat consumed and breast cancer. According to Dr. Michelle Holmes of Harvard Medical School, the study's lead author, "Our research indicates it's highly unlikely that women who consume a low-fat diet are protected against breast cancer. Equally, it appears a high-fat diet also poses no increased risk for the disease."[8])

The executive director of Shape Up America!, Barbara Moore, formerly a hired gun at Weight Watchers, told the *Wall Street Journal* that she "warned Dr. Koop that he was misrepresenting" the *JAMA* study on which he based his 300,000 deaths claim. To no avail, evidently, for he continues to spread this misinformation on the grounds that "it will eventually be shown"[9] that obesity kills 300,000 Americans each year. (This is rather like asserting that men and women *have* traveled to Mars because eventually they *will* travel to Mars.) Frances Berg of *Healthy Weight Journal* added that "We can't just charge in with a scattering of ill-considered programs,"[10] but her voice did not carry: Ms. Berg will never get closer to the South Lawn of the White House than the average tourist.

(The absurdity of Bill Clinton ordering a war on fat was pointed out by National Public Radio commentator Daniel Pinkwater, a girthful fellow himself, who noted,

> the president is a fat man, only he's resisting it. . . . I've heard the Secret Service steers him away from greasy food, and I submit this may be the problem. I was looking at our leader on television, and I noticed something in his face. It was an expression I had seen before. What was it, and where had I seen it? I remembered. I had seen it in my own face in the days before I accepted my glorious globular destiny. It was the expression of cheeseburger deprivation, calorie craving, schmaltz starvation. This man needs a french fry fix. Mr. President, eat something quick. I remember when I was on a diet. I made a lot of bad decisions. You owe it to our country to order the double pizza deal. We need you at your best. You can't do right unless you feel right.[11]

Not to worry, Mr. Pinkwater: Bill Clinton resisted very few temptations over the next few years.)

Koop himself, it must be noted, avoids cheeseburger deprivation. As Surgeon General Koop weighed in at a solid 6'1", 210 pounds. This is a perfectly reasonable height and weight: a tad on the overweight side, perhaps, but nothing to worry about. Or at least it didn't used to be.

Not that he's a beanpole. He grew his beard, he has said, to disguise hints of corpulency. "There were three chins," on his face, says Koop. "I said, 'No one is going to see those again.'"[12]

As Surgeon General he skipped lunch—"I'm too busy,"[13] he declared with typically inflated self-importance. His diet, by his own admission, teems with cholesterol. Macadamia nuts dipped in Cool Whip got him through many an operation back when he performed salutary work, and as he passed into the ranks of the elderly he took the eminently sensible position that "When you get to my age, you don't have to worry about blood levels or anything, because you've already proven you can beat the odds."[14]

While surgeon general, he was so heavy that he needed knee surgery. By his own admission, he lost fifteen pounds and the symptoms disappeared. Yet . . .

* * *

Just what exactly is Shape Up, America!? Located, in an amusing irony, on Democracy Boulevard in suburban Bethesda, Maryland, SUA! is a 501(c)(3) nonprofit "which receives a substantial part of its support from a governmental unit or the general public."[15] It takes in about $2.5 million annually, and these are not in $5 and $10 amounts from a grateful general public. For SUA! is, above all, a money-machine. Those corporations that stand most to benefit from an America panicky about a few extra pounds bought "Olympics-style sponsorships" of SUA!: Johnson & Johnson, Kellogg, good old Jenny Craig. In all, SUA! was propped up by thirty corporate sponsors. Most ignominiously, they included Wyeth-Ayerst of Redux infamy, NutriSystem, and Weight Watchers, whose agents infest the leadership of SUA! in the way that the mob once dominated the Teamsters. (No slight intended: James Hoffa the Younger has, we are sure, made that venerable union as pure as the plow-driven snow.)

Do we exaggerate? Consider this: every single one of the five staff members listed on the Shape Up America! roster was associated with Weight Watchers and/or H.J. Heinz, which manufacturers the "food" that Weight Watchers sells. This is beyond simple co-optation: even the Communists used to be more circumspect when setting up front groups. Starting at the top (after Koop, that is, who is as distant as the Olympian peak), we have Barbara J. Moore, president and CEO, who served as "General Manager of Program Development and primary technical policy advisor for Weight Watchers International." Next down the SUA! diet-food chain is Dr. William D. McArdle, a professor of Family, Nutrition, and Exercise Sciences (exercise sciences?) at Queens College of the City University of New York. Dr. McArdle's SUA! title is Nutrition and Exercise Consultant; he is "currently a member of the Scientific Advisory Board of Weight Watchers International." Then comes technical consultant Dr. Idamaria Laquatra, a dietician unlikely to gainsay the myriad qualities of ketchup: she was a nutritionist for Heinz USA and manager of nutrition services for Weight Watchers Food Company. She went on to serve as Vice President of Scientific Affairs and Training for Diet Center, Inc., a weight-loss franchise. Food Consultant and Cyberchef Lisa Schroeder is the next course: she developed and directed the nonfood products division (the better-tasting stuff) for Weight Watchers International. Last on the list is project manager Carol J. Morton, a former senior manager for Weight Watchers who "was responsible for the design and development of the psychological, exercise and service components of the Weight Watchers program."[16] For all intents and purposes, SUA! may as well call itself a subsidiary of Weight Watchers International.

Shape Up America! has all the commercial subtlety of the typical stock-car driver. But we are being too hard on the driver: He may be plastered over with patches for Valvoline and Michelin, but he does not pretend that these products are somehow essential to a good and long life. By contrast, when a boilerplate-filled flier called the *Eater's Almanac* is printed by Shape Up America! and Kellogg's Special K (a fast-fading cereal desperately in need of a jump-start) and developed by Giant Food, Inc., the implication is that Giant and Special K are part of the regimen of the shaped-up. Given that Giant sells, in addition to Special K, beer, cigarettes, potato chips, tater tots, fettucini alfredo, high-fat Ben and Jerry's ice cream, artery-clogging sausage, and aisle after aisle of food and liquid refreshment that give heart attacks to the nutrition nazis, if not to sated consumers, one might wonder just what the flagship organization of C. Everett Koop is doing in this company.

"Sponsorships" of SUA! are available to whichever company is willing to shell out the cash. It welcomes "food and beverage manufacturers, food retailers and restaurants, commodity boards, weight management companies, manufacturers of diet-related products [note how the previous two are slipped into the middle of the list], manufacturers of sporting goods and equipment, fitness organizations, health promotion companies and the mass media."[17] It doesn't matter if you make footballs or fajitas, diet pills or barbells: Dr. Koop Wants You!

The list of SUA!'s corporate sponsors is long, revealing, and occasionally amusing. *Time* magazine, soon to be the victim of Koop's video folly, gave Shape Up America! eight free pages in its May 8, 1995 issue: this amounted to $1.2 million in unpaid advertising. A leading candidate for the pharmaceutical hall of shame, Wyeth-Ayerst, marketer of Redux and the parent company of A.H. Robins, which marketed fen-phen, gave Shape Up America! and its even more grossly compromised sister organization, the American Obesity Association, $100,000 to publish "Guidance for Treatment of Adult Obesity," a set of guidelines for doctors who treat obesity. The document came out with great fanfare at a press conference presided over by Dr. Koop in October 1996 and aired live on CSPAN; his eminence granted interviews to ABC's "Good Morning, America," CNN, MSNBC, and Fox Morning News. More than 175 stories about the press conference were aired on stations across the country.

The big news, as *Health News Daily* headlined its article, was "Redux, Pondimin among Pharmacologic Therapies Recommended for Obese Patients."[18] About a year later, following the deaths of dozens of users of those pills Koop was pushing, Redux and Pondimin (one half of fen-phen), the drugs were pulled from the market. The advice given by America's doctor may have helped kill more patients than Dr. Jack Kevorkian and his suicide machine.

But let's face it: $100,000 is $100,000, and who but a saint or ascetic monk could turn down that kind of money? When the FDA approved Redux, SUA! honcho Barbara Moore gave it her seal of approval, saying that it's "not a magic bullet"[19] but nevertheless a real advance in weight control. Given the subsequent history of this killer drug, Moore's imprimatur seems to be at odds with SUA!'s stated goal of "providing credible, science-based health messages in a distinctive new way."[20]

The SUA!-AOA guidelines also recommended a variety of diets and even surgery, bringing smiles to the faces of a nation's bariatricians. Go ahead: call us witch doctors now; we've got the *Surgeon General of the United States* on our side! In a show of gratitude, the *American Journal of Bariatric Medicine* devoted the cover of its Fall 1996 issue to Dr. Koop, using artwork that so tickled him that it was reproduced in Shape Up America!'s annual report. "C. Everett Koop Declares War on Obesity,"[21] ran the caption over a cartoon of Koop, clad in combat fatigues, cradling a rifle, standing on an Iwo Jima-like island labeled "obesity," the American flag in the background. Once again, the war-avoiding Koop gets to don the khaki of fighting men in one of those metaphorical wars he so loves: the kind in which warriors don't get killed but American liberties do.

Needless to say, SUA! "developed important alliances with a number of federal government agencies,"[22] according to its annual report: it worked hand in glove on various tax-consuming projects with the Centers for Disease Control and Prevention, the White House Office of Science and Technology, the National Task Force on the Prevention and Treatment of Obesity, the National Institutes of Health Development, and the U.S. Department of Agriculture. Nevertheless, Koop insists that his plan was to "mount a privately funded anti-obesity initiative with the goal of incorporating many of the same strategies that the federal government has used so successfully to promote smoking cessation."[23] Endless hectoring, misuse of statistics, a ceaseless propaganda barrage, legal prohibitions, the omnipresence of the Koop face, scowling from the heights like Big Brother: the strategy seems better pitched to 1984 than 2000. But there is a twist: the funding is overwhelmingly private—that is to say, corporate—whereas the anti-smoking crusade is waged with money forked over by the hapless taxpayer, smoker or not.

The embattled Kellogg USA Inc. of Battle Creek, Michigan, determined to get the most bang for its million buck contribution to SUA!. It plastered the front of its boxes of Special K cereal with the SUA! logo: a silhouette of the forty-eight mainland states impressed with "Shape Up America!" and surrounded by "Founded by C. Everett Koop*Healthy Weight for Life." But that's not all. The back of the box, which in a sane world is devoted to hawking gimcracks and baubles to kids in exchange for seventy-three box tops of the product, is wholly devoted to the important announcement that "Kellogg's Special K and Shape Up America! [with trademark labels] have teamed up to announce a blend of vitamins and minerals which are important to help you stay healthy and strong." It goes on to list, in less than mouthwatering detail, the vitamins and minerals and acids contained in this modest box of cereal: a virtual passkey to eternal life, it seems. Shape Up America! denies that it endorses products, but "teamed up to announce a blend . . . " is so close to an endorsement that only the most lawyerly Jesuitical Clintonian could tell the difference. In any event, Kellogg's is not violating a trust: SUA! says that its sponsors and partners "are encouraged to use the logo,"[24] probably just as long as their contributions stay current. And while SUA! recommends that you eat "a bowl of cereal and wheat toast" for breakfast, it doesn't say *which* cereal. Okay, so the SUA! logo is all over the Special K box; still, Dr. Koop never comes right out and *says* to eat Special K. Wink, wink.

Do you recall Koop's boast early on in his career as a paragon of rectitude that he was offered a cool million to endorse a cereal but turned it down? After the Special K deal, he had best not trot out that line again.

Other sponsors range from the reputable to the shoddy. MET-Rx, a health supplement company, published SUA!'s booklet "99 Tips for Family Fun." Campbell's Soup has been a major backer of Shape Up America!—read the label of a typical Chunky soup and you'll find that it supplies about half the recommended daily allotment of saturated fat. Campbell's Soup also supplies canned food to Jenny Craig—good old Jenny, which basked in the reflected sunlight of Koopism. No company was more enthusiastic about Shape Up America! than Jenny Craig. Long disparaged as mountebanks taking advantage of the pudgy and the vulnerable, Jenny Craig was a like a trollop taken home by the prince to meet the royal family in the castle; she could not believe the company she was suddenly keeping. Hillary Clinton, C. Everett Koop; Jenny Craig even took to using the Shape Up America! logo—the forty-eight states, not a silhouette of a fat guy watching television—on its stationery. "We want the Shape Up America! logo to be as common as the logo for the Olympics,"[25] announced Koop.

Jenny Craig kicked in $1 million over SUA!'s first three years in the form of a "nonrestrictive grant," the type of grant one gives when one is confident that it will be put to a congenial use. The company played the Koop card for all it was worth. Jenny herself took to the air, blaring that her namesake "proudly sponsors"[26] Shape Up America! And by the way, as a means of sharing that pride, she offered a free week's worth of diet food to those willing to give Jenny Craig a try. Somewhere, the Campbell's Soup boy broke into an even wider version of his famous grin.

Jenny and Chick danced the K Street Waltz. He flew to Los Angeles to speak to 200 Jenny Craig franchise owners and employees. But this was renewing an old friendship, for in 1991 Dr. Koop came to San Diego to a salute to Sid and Jenny featuring such fading luminaries of the show-biz and mail-order magazine worlds as Ed McMahon and former *Eight is Enough* dad Dick Van Patten. It wasn't Morgan Fairchild, but a dim star beats no star at all.

In press releases, Jenny Craig repeated every absurd Koop claim, every hyperbolic statistic, every call for "a massive public education campaign that puts weight control into a different context for Americans so they are motivated to make change."[27] Experts and catalysts and clearinghouses and Change, always Change: Jenny Craig was thrilled to talk the same talk as the great Dr. Koop.

C. Joseph LaBonte, president and CEO of Jenny Craig, declaimed, "With an estimated 58 million adult Americans overweight, Jenny Craig is aware of the important role it will play augmenting Dr. Koop's efforts to educate Americans on the importance of achieving and maintaining a healthy body weight. . . . We have complete faith and confidence in Dr. Koop and his mission, and Jenny Craig will help in every way we can to make Shape Up America! a complete success."

Mr. LaBonte's confidence was well-placed. For if SUA! were a "complete success," our nation of tele-watching tubbies would break down the doors of every fitness center in America. Koop demanded a "national mobilization" against fat. His five-point national action plan was music to the ears of the diet industry: he called for "public education" efforts, which the less generous might call propaganda; insurance and workplace incentives for weight loss; "increased funding" for fitness and nutrition programs; greater physician involvement in weight loss and obesity prevention; and "significant increases" in federal spending on obesity research.[28] The federal budget, unlike the rest of us, was encouraged to swell and swell and swell. (Although Shape Up America! predicts that its "ultimate goal of stimulating behavior change" will lead to a "reduced demand for health care services"—including, presumably, weight-loss services—we may take this with a mountain of salt: it reminds us of the old Marxist claim that the state was to wither away after a brief but necessary totalitarian interlude.)

Despite its jaw-dropping conflicts of interest, Shape Up America! received a virtually free pass from the self-declared watchdogs (in practice, yuppie pups who can be mollified with a press release chew toy) of the mass media. Almost the only voice dissenting from the chorus of praise showered on the Chick and Hillary Show came from Lee Martindale in the *Dallas Morning News*, who asked the questions that lazy and complacent reporters did not:

> Shape-Up America! began with million-dollar donations from, among others, Jenny Craig, WeightWatchers and NutriSystem. Subsequent financial support has been provided by Wyeth-Ayerst, the American manufacturer of Redux, and the American Obesity Association, whose members primarily are weight-loss surgeons and bariatric specialists. I would think someone at least would suggest a link between the source of those donations and Dr. Koop's newest guidelines advocating dieting, very-low-calorie dieting, diet drugs and weight-loss surgery.
>
> When political campaigns use unsupported statistics, unfounded allegations and "facts" that are 180 degrees out of phase with the truth, we challenge them. When there is even a hint of special-interest influence, we call it what it is. We at least give the other side a chance for rebuttal. The fact that we don't treat "Shape Up America!" the same way is an indicator of how pervasive weight prejudice is. . . . [29]

And, she might have added, just how thoroughly Koop's carefully crafted reputation has hoodwinked potential critics and given him a free pass through the Garden of Cashing In.

A Shape Up America! Special Advertising Feature, produced for placement in magazines, provides a "hint of special-interest influence," to use Martindale's phrase, that is so obvious as to stun even the most doltish detective. On the very first page, before SUA! gets down to business, it gets down to its *real* business: a glossy full-page ad blazoned "Shape Up America! With Ultra Slim*Fast. . . . " Yes, the shake that kept Tommy Lasorda as round as a baseball is "a proud sponsor of the C. Everett Koop Foundation's Shape Up America! Campaign." The ad copy is, well, ad copy: barely edible food products are "tasty," "delicious," "fruity," and "luscious." They're "great for breakfast, lunch, sports, or any busy time." (Just ask Tommy!)

Next comes two pages of text under the menacing photo of Dr. Koop. "You believed me when I told you to quit smoking," he begins an ungrammatical sentence: the verb ought to be "obeyed," but that connotes coercion, submission, and other un-American acts. "I'm back with another warning," declares Koop: "smoking kills, but so does being overweight and inactive." Statistics follow, some accurate, some not. A lengthy biographical paragraph helpfully informs us of the ex-surgeon general's "pre-eminent" role in this and that. A photo of Koop and Mrs. Clinton—he's talking, she's listening—lets us know that he's still a Player.

After this we break for another full-page ad, this time for Kraft Fat Free Ranch Dressing. [Digression: The tobacco industry infiltrated this Koop-fest—Kraft is owned by a Big Tobacco company. But, hey, it helped to pay the bills.] A fitness quiz follows; it is slightly less sophisticated than the "Test Your Love Quotient" and "Do You Know How to Turn Him On?" exams found in the likes of *Cosmopolitan*. The knowledge that fitness "increases your self-esteem" is imparted a couple of pages later, just before an ad for Edge Extra Moisturizing Gel. This is a puzzler, though over the years the accumulated weight of hair shavings must add up, and who are we to criticize official sponsors of the national mobilization on fat? Photos of bike riders and a jogger remind us to "Get Up and Go" on the next page, but these are followed by a somewhat less taxing alternative: Hoffmann-LaRoche's ad for vitamin supplements. Why run when you can swallow?

The supplement concludes with food pyramid boilerplate sandwiched—wafered might be the better term here—around a full-page ad, with an American flag flying as backdrop, declaring "A healthy America starts with a healthier you." Brought to you by the good Australians of Jenny Craig. A picture of an uncharacteristically grinning C. Everett Koop standing with a beaming Jenny is in the center of the ad, surrounded by this text: "For over ten years, the idea of achieving and maintaining a healthy body weight has been the very heart of the Jenny Craig philosophy. So when C. Everett Koop told us about his Foundation's effort to teach Americans the value of weight loss, nutritional eating and exercise, it was music to our ears. Jenny Craig is proud to sponsor the C. Everett Koop Foundation and Shape Up America! So let's get together and go for it. What have you got to lose?"[30] (Beside your last shred of credibility, Dr. Koop?)

Note well that Jenny Craig claims that Koop approached them. In some cities this is called solicitation, but not, alas, in Washington.

Jenny Craig and Weight Watchers are getting their money's worth. Shape Up America! is always on the lookout for the barest shreds of evidence that weight-loss programs work. For instance, in October 1997 SUA! flooded the nation's newsrooms with a press release titled, "Study Finds Weight Loss Can Be Maintained; Provides New Hope to Overweight Americans." Now, this finding contradicted a virtual library's worth of previous research, which has conclusively determined that the weight that comes off in the early months goes back on. The principal investigator of the study, which was published in the

Journal of the American Dietetic Association—not quite a neutral site—conceded that the sample of twenty-two adults was very small. Too small, he did not say, to prove much of anything. These overweight adults were taught various "coping skills" that enabled them to maintain weight loss for two years—too short a time to establish the effectiveness of the treatment.[31] (Five years is the standard time line.) Nevertheless, SUA! responded as though life had been discovered on Mars. The study "offers hope that there may be practical and cost-effective approaches to obesity treatment that can be used in a variety of settings," gushed Barbara Moore. Such as a Jenny Craig center, she did not add.

The SUA! organized a Shape Up America! coalition of nonprofits to spread its message. Members ranged from the usual "nonprofit" suspects—the American Cancer Society, the American Association of Retired Persons, the American Medical Association—to the charlatans of the diet-drug front group the American Obesity Association to the—horrors!—hamburger-pushers of the National Cattlemen's Beef Association to such worthy, but seemingly out-of-place, groups as Harlem RBI (Reviving Baseball in Inner Cities).

Koop's pronouncements in the early years of SUA!, before more lucrative pastures beckoned, were full of his characteristic bluster, gross exaggeration, and stentorian hype. Obesity was a "crisis," naturally, and the bloated state of the American waist was "intolerable." We had grown fatter and fatter over the last 15 years, he harrumphed, seemingly not mindful of the implication that the surgeon general for a majority of those years must have been nodding off at the switch.

He took swipes at physicians, who "can no longer sit on the sidelines as America's obesity epidemic reaches crisis levels"[32]—a silly line, but give him credit for squeezing "crisis" and "epidemic" into the same sentence. To SUA!, obesity was "the disease that no one likes to talk about,"[33] an odd claim given the forests of trees felled each year to supply paper for the thousands of diet books published to meet the apparently ravenous public appetite for talk about obesity.

From the same deep well of absurdity out of which he had fished his 300,000 deaths Koop came up with this whopper: "If you eliminate just one of the three telephones in your house, you'll walk an extra 70 miles a year." *Seventy* miles a year? Perhaps if you live in William Randolph Hearst's San Simeon, and you have to run at a brisk jog to pick up the phone on fifteen rings.

But the phone was nothing in the creation of fat as compared with the television. The boob tube was the equivalent of having a French restaurant in the living room. It had a "significant influence on the development of obesity"[34] in children; in other words, TV causes disease! This is true no matter what the show, we assume: you're not getting any slimmer watching a C. Everett Koop video on angina. But while "TV is the no. 1 culprit . . . working at your computer is almost the same"[35]—this from a man who was soon to make millions pushing his own web site. Sometimes you wonder: is he even *aware* of the gross hypocrisy?

The workplace came in for special condemnation. The information age has meant "less physical activity on the job," as a nation of paper-pushers and pencil-sharpeners grows fatter by the clock-watched hour. (If only they could work as hod-carriers or coal-shovelers . . . now, those guys were in *shape*!) SUA! produced a guide to workplace fitness, *Fitting Fitness In, Even When You're Pressed for Time*, which was distributed, oddly enough, by the National Cattlemen's Beef Association. Working ranchers are unlikely to be uplifted by such advice as "In safe areas, par[k] your car at the back, or on the lowest level, of the garage or parking lot to increase your walk or climb."[36]

As usual, Founding Father Koop of SUA! displayed equal parts arrogance and political ineptitude. Consider his remarks about doctors and obesity. At a Shape Up America! news conference on October 30, 1996—a day later would have been more appropriate, given the good doctor's scare-hell-out-of-'em strategy—Koop predicted that SUA!'s propaganda "will literally change the way physicians think about obesity, from a vanity not discussed to a health-risk where physician intervention can actually save lives."[37]

Put aside, for the moment, the debate over the obesity-mortality link. Let's take Koop's words as gospel. (Though from all available evidence he regards himself as more the subject of the gospels than a mere writer of them.) How can it be that obesity is such a medical disaster and yet physicians think about it as simply a "vanity"? Is our medical profession really this far gone in cluelessness? If so, don't we *really* have serious problems as a nation with our incompetent health-care providers? Should the American people be launching an unprecedentedly massive class-action lawsuit against the country's army of malpracticing doctors? Does Koop understand the implications of his rhetoric? Or is he the only competent doctor in town—America's doctor, indeed?

Despite its millions in corporate subvention, Shape Up America! shared the fondness of its founder for the public teat. Among its earliest activities was the production of a series of twenty-, thirty-, and sixty-second "public service"—i.e., propagandistic—TV ads. They featured the familiar scowling phiz of C. Everett Koop warning of the evils of obesity (and gratuitously swiping at tobacco as well). The goal, admitted SUA! in its annual report, was "getting extensive unpaid air time": in other words, a public subsidy. A freebie. And it succeeded. In the first three months of the TV campaign, Shape Up America! got $3 million worth of "free" air time.

And what did SUA! achieve with this $3 million of TV time? By its own admission, 10,600 persons called the toll-free number listed in the ads for more information about obesity-related subjects.[38] That's 10,600 out of the 50 million—60 million, 70 million; it rises by the hour—Americans who are overweight. Do the math. We'll do the math ourselves in dividing $3 million by the 10,600 viewers who bothered to call what SUA! dramatically referred to as The Hotline. That comes to $283 per caller—a mighty expensive brochure. But hey, Koop got it free.

Shape Up America!, as a nonprofit 501(c)(3), is strictly limited in its ability to lobby the government. Its tax status, its very existence, depends on its refraining from pushing for or agitating against specific legislation. But many 501(c)(3)s skirt the line, confident that the Internal Revenue Service has better—or should we say worse—things to do than harass deep-pocket organizations. SUA!'s own material advertises its goal of "Informing Americans and Motivating Them to Act,"[39] and they don't just mean a brisk jog at dawn followed by a crispy bowl of Special K and a little red pill. The organization's website boasts that it is "advocating increased funding for school and community-based physical activity and nutrition programs."[40] Elsewhere, Shape Up America! urges such government actions as:

- "Expand community programs that promote physical activity"
- "Make physical education mandatory in schools" ("Mandatory," now *there*'s a Koop word)
- "Eliminate the deterrent of potential lawsuits by passing 'hold harmless' legislation for school physical education directors and teachers"
- "Provide childcare facilities in community recreation facilities"—"free child care," that is, while mom and dad pump iron or take an indoor walk rather than a family walk
- "Elevate walking as a national priority"

There is more, but the heart patients among our readers may have a hard time taking it all in: what a breathtakingly revolutionary agenda! Some of this is perfectly unobjectionable, even praiseworthy; some is, well, typically Koop. What seems undeniable is that such advocacy—SUA! organized a coalition to push for its policy proposals—violates the spirit of the tax code, which forbids a 501(c)(3) from promoting any particular piece of legislation. (You've probably seen the ritual disclaimers at the bottom of think-tank publications to the effect that nothing contained herein should be construed as encouraging blah blah blah. It's hogwash, and everyone knows it, but then the tax code is an animal product even more aromatic than hogwash.)

The preceding examples were taken from Koop's "10-step action plan" for physical activity. In pursuit of that nice round number, Koop and staff had to resort to such filler as "Mobilizing the nation's physicians to promote physical activity" and "Improving the safety of parks, sidewalks and recreational areas"[41] (Yes! *Crime* is now a physical fitness issue).

Shape Up America! also helped organize the Congressional Prevention Coalition (CPC), and with a name like that you know it's not dedicated to the defense of individual liberty. Koop spoke at the February 1998 Washington news conference that kicked off the CPC: he surveyed the landscape and found all sorts of candidates for prevention, from smoking to drinking to eating the wrong things. SUA! sponsored the first official activity of the CPC: a "Know Your Body Mass Index" screening for congresspeople and their staffs. The coalition's purpose, in the words of Senator John Chafee (R-RI), is to "focus on the ways in which we can prevent Americans from getting sick, rather than just rely on the tried-and-true methods of treating illness once it occurs." There was much talk of "investing" (spending tax dollars), "providing incentives" (coercing), and "educating"[42] (propagandizing). An ounce of prevention, it seems, is going to cost us a great deal of tax money and freedom. (Besides Chafee, the other founders of the CPC are Senator Bob Graham [D-FL] and Representatives James Leach [R-IA] and Jim Moran [D-VA].)

To the Koops of the world, liberty is fraught with danger: people will misuse the freedom to eat, the freedom to smoke, the freedom to supersize their french fries. So the feds must "identify individuals at risk for obesity,"[43] according to Shape Up America!, "and help them permanently alter their behavior to improve their health." If this sounds like the creation of an FBI-FDA data base tracking candy-bar eaters and Budweiser drinkers, then you must be an ultra-right-wing paranoiac. If SUA!'s call for "effective community interventions to promote healthful eating and increased physical activity"[44] sounds like mandatory jumping jacks, then you probably belong to a militia. If the constant calls for "increased funding" of this and that sound wasteful and intrusive, then you, good sir or madam, are mean-spirited and hateful. Relax: C. Everett Koop knows what's good for you.

As with many Beltway operations, Shape Up America! likes to commission polls to find what The Folks Out There are thinking. One SUA! survey polled public attitudes toward exercise—an innocuous, if not worthless, venture. A more comical poll reported that 70 percent of overweight American women have a "negative body image," as compared to 41 percent of thin women. We say "comical" because the survey was conducted for the Teresa and H. John Heinz III Foundation[45]—in other words, by the foundation set up by the folks who brought you Weight Watchers. The release of the results was accompanied by the usual bleating about stigmas and unattainable body images and self-esteem, with nary an acknowledgement that the diet industry has played a major role in encouraging women to be ashamed of the flesh that hangs on their bones. Perhaps the really startling number in this poll was the 41 percent of thin women who are unhappy with their bodies: this is the pool from which bulimics and anorexics are drawn.

Another survey found that 78 percent of obese and overweight Americans "are currently not on a diet," which must have made for a dark day at Weight Watchers. The "persistent anti-diet sentiment" was a cause for much grousing and grumbling at SUA!, but is it really all that mysterious a matter? One hundred percent of Americans love to eat, food is relatively cheap, and so the collective gut grows. What else is new? Nevertheless, SUA! insists that "the public is anxious for new materials that will help them learn how to achieve and maintain a healthy weight"—a proposition that is credible only if the SUA! survey is balderdash. Throughout SUA! materials there is a bizarre inconsistency between the alleged desires of Americans for information and their stubborn refusal to act on the voluminous information that SUA! and the federal government is shoveling toward them every day. "This anti-diet sentiment is very disturbing and provides a renewed sense of urgency that educating Americans about weight control cannot wait," declares Koop, but the dummies just won't take the hint. Which is why the hint will eventually become the prod if the nutrition nannies have their way. (SUA! noted that the reluctance to cut calorie intake "exists across the board among overweight individuals, regardless of educational attainment."[46] This includes, though the group does not note the fact, the 210-pound founder of SUA!.)

The whiff of preposterousness surrounded yet another SUA! poll, which purported to find that "poor people face major obstacles to exercise." As the *Los Angeles Times* reported, Shape Up America!'s Barbara Moore argued that "a lack of opportunity to exercise" is a prime reason that, paradoxically, the poor are fatter than the rich in the United States. Just why the poor are prohibited from, say, a workout at home or a walk around the neighborhood, she did not explain; she did note, however, that 46.5 percent of families earning less than $25,000 "felt they could not afford recreational facilities,"[47] which also begs a "yes, but" answer. Does walking, which SUA! quite rightly promotes as the best exercise of all, require "recreational facilities"? Another silly poll found that one-third of urban residents "indicated that child-care responsibilities limit their ability to get exercise."[48] Come again? Any parent will tell you that the triathlon is a breeze compared to raising a two-year old. "Child-care responsibilities" *require* exercise. As do such home tasks as washing, ironing, taking out the garbage, vacuuming; the list goes on. Do the folks at Weight Watchers—er, Shape Up America!—really think that the parents of toddlers have to go to community centers to get a workout? Please! Earth to Koop, Earth to Koop . . . (Come to think of it, Dr. Koop has confessed that in his single-minded devotion to career advancement, he neglected his own family, leaving the raising of his children to his wife, the smoke-free Betty.)

We have nothing against walking: indeed, we have done it all our lives. Shape Up America! is absolutely right to advise people to take the stairs rather than the elevator, and to get out for a walk now and then instead of sitting in front of the idiot box twelve hours a day. But in its bid to darken the whiter than white hue of the nutrition-fitness complex, SUA! goes to absurd, patently patronizing lengths to demonstrate its commitment to the right of people of color to take a walk. The "biggest challenge" he faces, Koop said, straight-facedly, is "letting people know that physical activity is something everyone can do."[49] It *is*?!

Dr. Koop asserts that "obesity is not an equal opportunity disease": donuts, evidently, shun wealthier eaters and plot and scheme to make their way into the tummies of the poor. The disadvantaged also have "more difficulty adding fruits and vegetables to their diet"—why, we are not told, beyond a false claim that they cost more than junk food. "Lower-income Americans are at a greater risk for obesity because they lack the resources that many of us take for granted," he continues, urging "community action" to "make it easier for those with a lower income to adopt a healthier lifestyle."[50] Just what form might this "community action" take? Nothing quite as benign as, say, government-issued, means-tested vouchers for the purchase of Stair Masters. Rather, we are to help the poor by depriving them of the right to make unhealthy choices: virtually ban cigarettes, restrict alcohol sales and advertising, and, ultimately, tax fatty foods so as to make them unaffordable for all but the country-club set. The $10-a-package Ho-Ho will acquire new cachet: formerly skeletal ladies in the horsy set will compete in the adipose sweepstakes. Obesity will become an equal opportunity condition—oh, all right, "disease"—and the p.c. police will rest easier in the knowledge that cellulite is no longer the exclusive curse of the starving class.

In any event, tribunes of the poor will be overjoyed to know that SUA! is involved in the Partnership for a Walkable America (PWA), which is "removing barriers to walking."[51] We are not, we assure you, making this up.

There is much in the SUA! agit-prop about "minority Americans and the medically-underserved," whose health is to be improved by "tailored and empowering messages."[52] These include the heretofore unknown facts that, in order to measure one's height, you must "Stand with your head, buttocks and feet touching a vertical wall" and "consistently consuming more energy (calories) than you burn will cause *weight gain* and burning more energy (calories) than you consume will cause *weight reduction.* It's really as simple as that!"[53] Now *that's* empowering! As is the knowledge that "moving more throughout the day is what is really important."[54] In fact, the unobjectionable parts of the SUA! program—which can be boiled down to (1) eat healthy food in reasonable portions; and (2) exercise—are not exactly rocket science. This is what Mom taught you when you were five years old.

Riding the p.c. rail, Dr. Koop and SUA! have also tried to frame obesity as a women's issue. "[W]omen are paying significantly higher costs for their obesity, both in terms of health expenditures and their quality of life,"[55] than men, reads one press release. Two-thirds of obesity-related doctor's office visits were made by women: good news for bariatricians, one would think. SUA! neglects to note the percentage of diet pill expenditures made by women (upwards of 90 percent), but then that appalling figure throws a different light on the issue. For it suggests that the scare-mongering, thin-worshipping hucksters of the diet and fitness industries have succeeded in conning women into buying the notion of Cindy Crawford as the ideal woman. The millions of anorexics and bulimics, also overwhelmingly women, do not compute either, for excessive thinness is as dangerous, if not more so, than obesity, but SUA! knows which end of the tap the money comes through.

"When it comes to obesity, women are truly disadvantaged," declares Weight Watchers functionary turned SUA! leader Barbara J. Moore. "Not only are they more likely to become immobilized by obesity than are men, but they become less able to run errands, buy groceries and lead independent lives."[56] Just why a 300-pound woman has a tougher time buying groceries than a similarly large man is not explained: wags may jest that staying away from the grocery store may not be all bad for the obese, but we can see Moore's point: anything that keeps a potential customer from buying Heinz products is an unmitigated evil.

Foreshadowing a later enthusiasm that would make Koop rich beyond the dreams of Croesus, Shape Up America! launched a CYBERKitchen. It didn't serve food, alas, but "information." You will recall that one of the endless Shape Up America! polls had found that overweight Americans were not getting with *the plan*: 78 percent of them had told pollsters that they were not dieting. This conflicts with most other polling data, which show Americans to be a diet-obsessed people, but no matter: either way, *something must be done*! For as a grave Dr. Koop intoned, "Until we give people the educational tools to fight obesity, they will remain frustrated and confused, and obesity will continue to skyrocket."[57] More to the point, Jenny Craig and Weight Watchers food will remain on the shelves, and we can't have that now, can we? So the misnamed CYBERKitchen, launched with a publicity blitzkrieg that got Koop free face-time on NBC's "Today" show, CNN, CNBC, Fox, and the TV Food Network, was designed for the handful of poor souls who cruise the net seeking "educational tools to fight obesity."[58] Just type in age, weight, height, and level of physical activity and shazam, the chefs at the CYBERKitchen will whip up your own personal daily calorie goal and throw in "healthful" recipes as well. Who could resist?

Again and again with Shape Up America!, the fault is said to lie with those chubby lamebrains who simply cannot get it through their thick skulls that THIN IS GOOD. People are "not dieting because they are confused,"[59] said Dr. Louis J. Aronne upon the opening of SUA!'s CYBERKitchen. Barbara Moore told an Indianapolis obesity seminar that "People need to figure out ways to be more physically active and learning [*sic*] the basics of portion control,"[60] knowledge that is usually gained by about the first grade.

Fat costs the country $100 billion a year, Moore threw in for good measure—a coincidentally round number, no? But here she was repeating a favorite Koop theme, and that old standby of the therapeutic state: the "cost to society" of obesity. The aggregate figures for the treatment of diabetes are this much, for heart disease that much, for breast cancer this much (oops: the breast-cancer obesity link has been discredited—make that colon cancer, at least for now). From out of thin air Koop pulls a figure of $45.8 billion in "direct costs," such as hospital and physician care. Add up indirect—which is to say, even less substantial—costs, throw in eye of newt and tongue of lizard, and at the end of all this computing we are presented with the bill for obesity: a staggering $100 billion-plus. Not to mention 53.6 million workdays per year lost to obesity.[61] The implication is that these inconsiderate lardasses are bankrupting the country, and therefore the rest of us, acting through the medium of the federal government, have the obligation to discipline them. This is much the same argument that the smoking prohibitionists make, always leaving aside the counterclaim that if smoking or obesity really do kill people prematurely, they function as net gains to the treasury because the deceased are not around to receive costly end-of-life care in their seventies, eighties, and nineties (not to mention their social security checks). Of course these utilitarian calculations are appalling no matter *what* they "prove": a person's life and liberty are not reducible to lines on a cost-benefit sheet. At least not to those who regard persons as distinct individuals and not mere heads in a herd.

"[I]s Shape Up America! making a difference?"[62] Dr. Koop asked two years and several million dollars into the venture. You bet it is! It smoothed the way for Redux and fen-phen. It repeated the 300,000 annual obesity deaths canard so frequently that it became an accepted factoid. By recommending "drug therapy" for the obese, it encouraged a pharmaceutical approach to weight loss, which pleases Koop's sponsors but has been dangerously ineffective in the past.

* * *

Every inflated statistic and half-baked claim comes together in the mission statement of the American Obesity Association: "Obesity is a disease that affects at least 70 million [up from Koop's 58 million] Americans; more than one-third of all adults and one in five children. . . . Each year, obesity causes at least 300,000 excess deaths in the U.S. and costs the country more than $100 billion."[63] Making the point as tastelessly as possible, American Obesity Association vice president Judith S. Stern told a congressional subcommittee that "premature deaths due to overweight equal over 4 Oklahoma City bombings a day."[64] Though Timothy McVeigh, at least, was lean.

The American Obesity Association (AOA) is a classic Washington, D.C. front group. Created in 1995, it is almost entirely subsidized by the pharmaceutical industry: such diet-drug makers and marketers as American Home Products, Interneuron, Roche Laboratories, Knoll Pharmaceuticals Ltd., and Servier. Cofounder Richard L. Atkinson "describes the AOA as a 'lay advocacy group' that is a 'vigorous new advocate' for the 70 million [70 million?] Americans who suffer from the disease of obesity."[65] Seventy million constituents! This number makes the AFL-CIO, NRA, AARP, and the rest of the alphabet-soup interest groups look like pikers. But, alas, though the group is for heavy members, it is not membership heavy. In one priceless paragraph in the *Wall Street Journal*, its investigative reporters found: "The Association charges individuals $25 for membership. [Cofounder] Dr. [Judith S.] Stern says she and Dr. Atkinson belong but she has 'absolutely no idea' how many others are members. Asked for a member count, Morgan Downey, the group's executive director, produced a single, completed application and said it was from the only paid member he had seen."[66]

The thought of this advocacy group, with its annual budget in the hundreds of thousands of dollars, lobbying and testifying and publishing, all for the sake of its one single solitary member, is enough to fill the most ruthless heart with pity. One member! The Gary Coleman fan club is bigger than that!

Dr. C. Everett Koop sits on the Advisory Council of the AOA; his colleagues include the notorious Dr. Xavier Pi-Sunyer, a man who thinks Cal Ripken, Jr. is dangerously overweight, and Barbara J. Moore, the Weight Watchers functionary turned Shape Up America! president. In an interesting editorial decision, Ms. Moore's years of toil for Weight Watchers are omitted from her biography in the AOA's portraits of its Advisory Council. This is a switch: usually in Washington, resume-*padding* is the problem, but with Ms. Moore, we have a case of resume-reduction. Or perhaps this is in keeping with the Weight Watchers' philosophy of irrational pound-shedding. Also on the council is Dr. G. Michael Steelman, the Oklahoma City-based president of the American Society of Bariatric Physicians. (Steelman also helped write the Shape Up America!-AOA "Guidance for the Treatment of Adult Obesity," as did Doctors Atkinson, Stern, and Barbara J. Moore.)

Koop's *ex cathedra* pronouncements on obesity—"a new epidemic," he calls it, but then what *doesn't* he call a new epidemic—are widely promulgated by the AOA. And why not? His alarmism, his use of inflated statistics, his willingness to make assertions unsupported by fact ("Among post-menopausal women, 11 percent of breast cancer is estimated to be attributable to obesity"[67]—flat untruth), his flacking for whichever corporation will pay him well: Koop fits in well at the American Obesity Association. "If I had been able to do one more thing during my tenure as Surgeon General," he says ruefully, "it would have been to launch a campaign against obesity."[68] Thank heavens for the four-year term.

President Atkinson and Vice President Stern are the public face of the American Obesity Association—though curiously, neither is obese, nor is anyone else on the advisory council.

"I know the AOA touts itself as a consumer group,"[69] Sally Smith, executive director of the National Association to Advance Fat Acceptance, told the *Wisconsin State Journal*, but "I don't believe they're a consumer group at all. Most of the people on the board of the AOA are on the payroll of the weight-loss industry."

Even in a town marked by a jaded acceptance of rented scholarship and hired intellectual guns, the American Obesity Association stands out. During the Redux/fen-phen controversy of the mid-1990s, Dr. Atkinson, a VMI graduate and head of the University of Wisconsin-

Madison's Clinical Nutrition Clinic, became the reassuring voice of the diet drug industry, insisting, "I'm not going to take a single person off fen-phen—unless they ask me to—because this [critical Mayo Clinic] study is not adequate."[70] Two months later, Atkinson's paymasters at Wyeth-Ayerst Laboratories and Interneuron Pharmaceuticals pulled fen-phen and its sister, Redux, from the market. Properly grateful for Atkinson's making a fool of himself, they did not pull funding from the AOA. For good measure, AOA executive director Morgan Downey said—with utter frankness and brutal honesty, we are sure—"It seemed to me that Wyeth-Ayerst acted quickly and responsibly in withdrawing its products when the Mayo data came to light."[71] (For more on fen-phen and the AOA, see the next chapter.)

Atkinson and Stern claim that they launched the AOA intending it to be something other than just another business-suited whore for corporate interests. "Our original plan was not to be beholden, like *Consumer Reports*," says Atkinson. "But that simply didn't work."[72] So they became beholden.

Atkinson's public remarks are music to the ears of the pharmaceutical companies. Back in 1994, when he was singing the praises of diet drugs ("New Diet Pills Under Study Win Praise From Obesity Expert," blared the headlines), Atkinson predicted that in the enlightened near future, obesity will be "just like hypertension. If you are unfortunate enough to have the genetic disease of obesity, you are going to have to take drugs the rest of your life."[73] Eureka! screamed Wyeth-Ayerst, which became a major supporter of the AOA. But then it was just returning a favor; Atkinson had reported in 1993 the early results of his own study of fen-phen: it "showed not only dramatic weight loss, but that his patients' cholesterol, high blood pressure and blood sugar levels dropped or returned to normal."[74]

Morgan Downey, executive director of AOA, doubted from the first that it could survive as a membership organization, for the very good reason that "I could not see myself with a bumper sticker that proclaimed, 'Proud Member, American Obesity Association.'"[75] Evidently, only one such person exists in all our land, that lonely fat-proud member whose application Downey waved at the *Wall Street Journal*. Instead, over 90 percent of the AOA's budget comes from corporate donors, who are thanked on occasion in the group's quarterly newsletter, the *AOA Report*. Wyeth-Ayerst, Interneuron, Knoll Pharmaceuticals, Thompson Medical, and Hoffman LaRoche Laboratories are prime sugar (Nutra-Sweet?) daddies.

In addition to its not-yet-filled-up general membership category, the AOA offers a variety of, shall we say, "unusual" memberships. Just $800 a year earns an Obesity Specialty clinic membership; shell out $3,000 and you'll be designated a Center of Excellence on Obesity (CEO). No, this does not mean that the designee has achieved excellence in obesity; say, a perfectly rounded corpulence. Rather, a CEO must have published three pieces (however mediocre) in peer-reviewed journals over the last five years or have taught "professional service providers to patients with obesity" at the graduate level. Behold . . . excellence!

Finally, for $5,000 a year the lucky applicant can be a "Corporation Providing Products for Patients with Obesity." The big-money donors are subject to the most rigorous possible scrutiny: their claims "may be subject to review and approval of AOA."[76] Oooh!

According to the AOA, it has about 500 dues-paying corporate "members." Virtually everything the AOA does is underwritten by the weight-loss industry; its putatively public-spirited "Weight Wellness Week" was paid for by Medeva Pharmaceuticals. And so Weight Wellness Week was no mere pep rally for workouts at the fitness gym and eating more fruits and vegetables; no, this "complex disease" of obesity was said to require "multi-faceted treatment." For "many patients [diet and exercise] are not enough, and medication may be required."[77] And please patronize our sponsors on your way out.

Executive director Downey makes the laughable claim that the AOA is motivated by the purest heart: "It wasn't a matter of being a shill for Wyeth-Ayerst," he said of the fen-phen flacking. "It was more, 'What's in the best interest of the patients who had very serious problems with obesity?'"[78]

Like his advisor Koop, Atkinson puts out for his contributors. When the FDA held a hearing on MERIDIA, Knoll Pharmaceuticals' big-ticket weight-loss drug, the good doctor testified . . . in favor of approval! This came just months after the fen-phen debacle; indeed, in the same issue of the *AOA Report* in which Morgan Downey was spinning AOA's shameful conduct in the matter of fen-phen, a headline hailed the "New Drug to Combat Obesity." It was MERIDIA, brought to rotund Americans by the Knoll Laboratories that helps subsidize the AOA. The *AOA Report* noted that Knoll would engage in "responsible marketing" of MERIDIA; it had even drawn up its own "ethical marketing credo,"[79] for goodness sake.

AOA members are expected to post the group's patient bill of rights, which mixes such bland claims as "Patients have the right to be treated with dignity and respect at all times" (as opposed to being addressed as "Mr. Fatass," we presume?) with highly debatable claims masked as axioms, such as "Patients have the right to know that obesity is a chronic health disease . . ." and "Patients have the right to know that being overweight or obese is a serious disease with known health risks."[80] (Of course, many non-diseases—riding motorcycles, hang-gliding—carry health risks as well.)

The AOA's 501(c)(4) designation permits it to lobby. Its "fundamental mission" is "to have obesity regarded for what it is—a disease of epidemic proportions."[81] And what is the best way to cure a disease? Federal funding, of course. There is no limit to the number of federal dollars that the obesity researchers of AOA believe should go toward obesity research. To themselves, in other words. "Research is severely limited by a shortage of funds,"[82] the AOA declares; indeed, the level of government support is "shockingly low," and this despite the "eloquent" dissertations on the cost of obesity by Dr. C. Everett Koop, whose pearls of wisdom are cast throughout AOA publications. AOA's initial demand: a "five-fold"[83] increase in government spending. At a joint AOA-SUA! press conference, Koop told the assembled journalists that NIH spending on obesity research was "minuscule" given the "epidemic" (ho-hum) nature of the "disease."[84]

"Urging health insurance payers, both governmental and private, to treat obesity as they do other major diseases"[85] is a prime goal of the AOA, and a clue to why its 1999 first quarter *AOA Report* lists Jenny Craig, Weight Watchers International, the American Society of Bariatric Physicians, and the American Society for Bariatric Surgery as "supporters." In 1998, Knoll Pharmaceutical Company sponsored publication of the AOA's *Weight Management and Health Insurance*, a booklet that complains, "Your health insurance company . . . may be reluctant to pay for the costs of your weight-loss treatment" and spends the next several pages urging readers "to make your needs known." Not only to the insurance company but, in the event of a rejection, to "state and federally elected officials who may be able to assist you in the appeals process."[86] Just why a U.S. Senator should play a role in an insurance company's decision whether to pay for, say, a MERIDIA prescription is a bit mysterious, though some might call it bullying.

Imagine, if you will, John Lennon-like, a world in which your insurance company is required by law to cover the cost of your Weight Watchers TV dinner, your cosmetic liposuction, your Redux prescription, your early morning fen-phen, your Jenny Craig consultation, your chat with a bariatric witch doctor . . . surely, this would be a just world, a sane world, a world in which people of all shapes and sizes could live together, in harmony, all hoping to eventually achieve the exact same shape and size, courtesy of the lobbying efforts of the American Obesity Association.

The AOA displays the trademark schizophrenia of the weight-loss hucksters: decrying "lookism" while not so subtly promoting the denigration of the chunky. "Our society as a whole is focused on looks—the thinner, the better—[*sic*] seems to be the thinking promoted by Madison Avenue," declares Richard Atkinson, sounding like a fat-acceptance guru. "This erroneous thinking has created a nation of people obsessed with their looks. Our children are growing up worried more about 'how thin' they are than how their characters are being molded." Right on, bulky brother—yet in the very same paragraph he warns, "You don't have to look FAT to be considered obese," and he goes on to detail the countless illnesses that afflict those who eat "tasty, high-fat foods" instead of the "fat substitutes and low fat foods"[87] recommended by the AOA. You can almost hear the ching! of the AOA cash register.

Atkinson has made a regular sideline of defending fat substitutes. In 1996, when the fat substitute olestra had just been cleared by the Food and Drug Administration and potato chips made therefrom were being test-marketed by Procter and Gamble in Cedar Rapids, Iowa; Grand Junction, Colorado; and Eau Claire, Wisconsin, Atkinson visited Cedar Rapids to urge the potato chip eaters of that city to ignore the "alarmist" claims of such Chicken Little groups as the Center for Science in the Public Interest (CSPI), which had dubbed the three cities the "diarrhea capitals" of America because of the alleged "fecal urgency" the chips produced in some consumers.

The CSPI claims were a joke, as we have argued in our book, *The Food and Drink Police: America's Nannies, Busybodies, and Petty Tyrants*.[88] The "gastrointestinal horror stories" adduced by the nannies of CSPI were no more horrific than the run-to-the-bathroom tales that could be told by every adult American. The unpleasant side effects of eating olestra-based chips were vastly overblown, if not spun out of whole cloth. But we did not write our book in the hopes of getting money from the makers of fat substitutes. (As a footnote, CSPI was spawned in the same Naderite pond that Morgan Downey once swam in. Torn asunder, it seems, by the politics of fecal urgency.)

Also high atop the AOA agenda is rewriting *Healthy People 2010*, our "national health charter." (We'll bet you didn't even know we had one. And by the looks of it, there is no chance that it might be retitled *Free People 2010*.) The decennial Healthy People series was a 1979 brainchild of the Surgeon General's office; thereafter, every ten years the people of the United States were to be harassed by the public health totalitarians. For instance, *Healthy People 2000* decreed that, come the millennium, no more than 20 percent of American adults and 15 percent of adolescents would be overweight. According to the government's statistics, that didn't happen. *You Americans didn't get with the program! Diet: Now! Or heads will roll! Healthy People 2000* also failed to talk down teen suicide rates: strangely, suicide attempts by teenagers increased during the 1990s, but suicide deaths did not.

Healthy People 2010 is a thick publication of the U.S. Department of Health and Human Services "aimed at increasing the quality and length of life." Yet, scandalously, the draft circulating in 1999 "virtually ignored obesity and its threat to national well-being." Unlike, say, heart disease and diabetes, obesity didn't even get its own chapter. To paraphrase President Bush, this could not stand. In the language of psychobabble, "It is time for the public health community to stop being in denial about obesity," AOA executive director Morgan Downey told the other members of the Healthy People Consortium. Now, just how the American Obesity Association qualifies for membership in the Healthy People Consortium is a bit of a mystery—unless the obese are healthy. Be that as it may, Downey demanded "a broad campaign" on every front "to stop this epidemic before it becomes the normative condition in the United States. We cannot wait for *Healthy People 2020* to address obesity."[89]

Healthy People 2010 was issued January 25, 2000 and, of course, contains health goals on obesity. All the usual hype is repeated, including the claim that obesity cost the nation $99 billion in 1995. Interested readers (or the terminally bored) may wade through the conventional wisdom at the internet site, www.health.gov/healthypeople/document.html/volume1/weight.htm.

Taking Koopism one step further, AOA insists that obesity is not just a disease, it is "a disability." Employment discrimination, social stigma, lack of access to attractive mates . . . the consequences of this disability are staggering. Government action is needed to Set Things Right.

So are more benign forms of thought control. The *AOA Report* rejoiced when the lexicographers at Merriam-Webster announced that they were considering the inclusion of the idiotic term "sizeism" in their dictionary. The term, used only on the furthest shores of the kingdom of the Politically Correct, is defined as "prejudice against people because of their size, especially when viewed as overweight or short." (NBA centers ought to sic their players' union on this one: isn't asking the 7'6" Shawn Bradley how the weather is up there a classic instance of sizeism?) The *AOA Report* also instructs readers on the correct way to deal with insensate brutes who note, say, that a 500-pound man is big: "If a biased comment is made in your presence, you would be grammatically correct to caution the speaker against becoming a sizeist."[90] This will do until such remarks are legally defined as hate speech, at which point the offender can be imprisoned for an appropriate length of time.

Jokes are *verboten* at AOA. The organization shifted into high dudgeon when the District of Columbia tried to loosen its definition of disability to include obese policemen. Congress oversees the district's affairs, and one member of that august body had the temerity to make his point with a joke: "Disability shouldn't be something that happens when you are 300 pounds and can't bend over to eat a doughnut." Morgan Downey was outraged: "It is inconceivable that a legislator would speak so contemptuously of people with diabetes, AIDS, or lung cancer."[91] Yes, it is. Because those, unlike obesity, are diseases.

(Maybe Downey should subject his colleague Koop to a sensitivity lesson. The doctor has complained, "Smokers are doing something that can be harmful to others, so you can say, 'This is a smoke-free house or business.' But when you say something about fat, people get their feelings hurt."[92] We suppose they would object to the establishment of a fatty-free house.)

Morgan Downey, perhaps the last man in American who can use the phrase "in denial" with a straight face, is the token fatso at AOA. Or should we say recovering fatso, to borrow the therapeutic jargon of the organization. A public-interest lawyer formerly with (the rail-thin) Ralph Nader and Common Cause, Downey was a subject in the George

Washington University Obesity Management Plan, a fact that AOA blares in its literature. "He knows obesity issues first hand,"[93] enthuses Richard Atkinson, with the boundless excitement of a 1960s suburban liberal who has just invited a real live actual Negro person to a party.

There is something creepy about the way Downey speaks of his weight. "I am a person with obesity," he testified, as if at an Alcoholics Anonymous meeting in the basement of the Methodist church. "It is in remission now, but before I started treatment I weighed over 250 lbs."[94] In *remission*? This is borderline offensive, talking about heft as though it were leukemia. He goes on to compare obesity to mental illness: in neither case is the condition the victim's "fault," but the stigma of obesity is even harsher than that of mental illness. You can guess where this is going: just as the last decade has seen a push to force insurers to cover treatment for mental illness—not just psychosis but your garden variety neurotic's weekly session with his shrink—so must treatment for obesity be covered. And if the AOA's corporate members would benefit greatly from such coverage: hey, life is full of coincidences.

To the AOA, every act, every moment, every thought in this world that does not lead to the immediate coverage of obesity treatment and the exponential expansion of federal obesity research is "shameful." Neglectful. Unconscionable. All those words that pad the thesauruses of Beltway publicists. As is often the case with weight-loss promoters, the AOA seems to be making almost constant puns on its mission, unintentionally, no doubt. Dr. Judith Stern appeared before the House Subcommittee on Labor, Health and Human Resources, and Education and Related Agencies to warn of the "growing epidemic"[95] of obesity. Yes, we guess obesity could be termed a growing epidemic, though this seems to contradict Dr. Atkinson's plea that we no longer regard the large as "the proper butt of jokes." Atkinson also pledges to mount a nationwide grass-roots campaign to press his agenda once his "membership is of sufficient size"[96]—at which point, presumably, the AOA's work would be done. Childhood obesity is also deemed a "growing problem"[97]: read enough of these and you wonder if some impish editor at the AOA isn't committing hate thought in the very belly of the beast itself.

Other AOA proposals include "a comprehensive plan to create healthy weight programs in schools"[98] and income tax deductibility for obesity-treatment expenses. There are, to be fair, perfectly innocuous materials issued under the group's name. "Sticking With It: How to Avoid Becoming an Exercise Dropout," contains reasonable recommendations for those who want to get in shape, but one gets the impression that Wyeth-Ayerst and Knoll don't want too many of their donated dollars going to exhort readers to "Work out to your favorite exercise video, play with your pet, or go walking at the mall with a friend."[99] That pabulum is okay as far as it goes, which isn't very far at all; more appropriate advice, given who is paying this particular fiddler, might be "Lay around, grouse about the unfairness of it all, write a letter to your congressman demanding more federal funding for obesity research, and pop a few weight-loss pills."

However absurd AOA may be, it has learned to play the public relations game. Its September 1999 conference on Obesity: The Public Health Crisis, held in Washington, DC, featured a continental breakfast hosted by Sarah Ferguson, the Duchess of Pork and Weight Watchers shill, who was not devouring donuts, at least not before the assembled nutrition nannies. Conference rhetoric was shrill: "While we have this two-day meeting, 1,800 people will be dead from problems related to obesity," shouted Dr. Judith Stern. "This is a national emergency."[100] And in a national emergency, the first casualties are American liberties. Among those draconian measures proposed at the AOA conference: slapping prohibitive taxes on fatty foods, increasing the school day so that students can engage in exercise right out of an old Nazi Youth handbook, and, of course, but of course, SPENDING MORE TAXPAYERS' MONEY.

In 1996 the AOA and what it calls its "sister" organization, Shape Up America!, teamed to produce "Guidance for the Treatment of Adult Obesity," the tone of which can be gathered from the remark by Dr. Patricia S. Choban of Ohio State University Medical Center, a writer of the report, who said, "We are talking about a disease. This is about your risk of dying."[101] A strange definition of disease, but then the ultimate success of the AOA and the corporations that subsidize it depends on the fear they can whip up among the citizenry. And as nothing scares people quite like death, death it is.

"Guidance for Treatment of Adult Obesity" begins, of course, with the asseveration, "Obesity is a disease . . . " and it doesn't get any better. (Is there another disease known to man that can be cured by pushing back from the dinner table?) Doctors are encouraged to "Examine your own feelings about obesity and the obese"[102] and to banish bad thoughts. Be supportive, listen, empathize, and, most importantly, agitate for obesity to be covered under private and governmental health insurance. With the AOA, SUA!, and Dr. C. Everett Koop, the punch line is always . . . send money.

But like graduates of a self-esteem school, they can live with that. "I get up in the morning and I look in the mirror and I feel good about myself,"[103] says Atkinson. Not because he is not fat—and besides, if he does put on a few pounds there are wonder drugs to take them right off again—but because he is selflessly serving the obese. (What they'd really like is a jelly donut. . . . Pardon the insensitivity. But it is impossible to read through volumes of hypocritical cant by thin shills for the drug companies masquerading as noble altruists without the occasional irreverent burst.)

* * *

Government health guidelines are notoriously fickle and about as stable as an Elizabeth Taylor marriage. For instance, neo-prohibitionists within the Departments of Agriculture and Health and Human Services once wrote the federal Dietary Guidelines for Americans (and just what is the constitutional basis of *that* activity?) to state that "drinking has no net health benefit." This was a bald falsehood: hogsheads of research had established that wine consumption is related to a lower incidence of heart disease. But the public health nannies shy from honesty on matters alcoholic as primitive man shied from fire. It wasn't until 1996 that the federal dietary guidelines admitted that "moderate drinking is associated with a lower risk for coronary heart disease." Throwing prudery to the wind, at least for the time being, the diet bureau even observed that "alcoholic beverages have been used to enhance the enjoyment of meals by many societies throughout human history."

(At least the diet mandarins grudgingly conceded the truth. C. Everett Koop's *Surgeon General's Report on Nutrition and Health* stood firm against the admission of even the slimmest ray of veracity. Marion Nestle, chair of the Department of Nutrition and Food Studies at New York University and the managing editor of the surgeon general's nutrition report, has described the report as "rather prohibitionist," a slant she attributes largely to "the Surgeon General himself, Dr. C. Everett Koop, a self-described evangelical Christian who viewed alcohol as an addictive drug. Dr. Koop has written, 'When we convince ourselves . . . to say 'No!' to drugs such as alcohol and nicotine, we take charge of our health' and 'alcohol is a toxic, potentially addictive drug, the greatest killer of America's youth.'" The martini-swilling surgeon general "was firmly opposed to allowing any statement in the report or recommendation that might even hint at any possible benefit of alcohol consumption."[104] So there you have it: the old hypocrite—a self-described *drug user*!—bars from the *Surgeon General's Report on Nutrition and Health* an honest discussion of the potential benefits of moderate alcohol consumption. This is a profile in something, but surely it is other than courage.)

The pleasure-quashers hold the upper hand in the agencies of the federal government. (Surprise!) Consider the efforts of a handful of sensible nutritionists to add to the U.S. Dietary Guidelines the truly revolutionary exhortation to enjoy eating. It was as if the Drug Enforcement Administration were asked to plaster "Coke Adds Life" to their propaganda brochures. A group called the International Food Information Council pointed out that the British, who are known neither for their delectable cuisine nor their unbuttoned style, begin their government dietary guidelines with the instruction, "Enjoy your food." The Norwegians suggest that "food and joy equal health." The Vietnamese—the Vietnamese, for crying out loud: commies!—tell their subjects to eat food "that is delicious . . . and served with affection." But when Eileen Kennedy, the Clinton administration deputy undersecretary for research, education, and economics within the Department of Agriculture, urged that the U.S. Dietary Guidelines be revised to read, "Enjoy a variety of foods,"[105] her fellow bureaucrats rejected it as "too hedonistic." To enjoy food, in the eyes of government officials, is tantamount to lounging by a pool with a bevy of starlets and case of champagne. It is positively decadent. The guidelines wound up advising us to "Eat a variety of foods": eat but don't enjoy. But then this was the administration of a president who reduced sex with a twenty-one-year-old intern to a joyless, mechanistic act.

Sometimes government health guidelines can have tragic fall-out. In June 1998, 29 million Americans became fat overnight. In May, 68 million Americans had been officially overweight—and many of them were living perfectly normal and healthy lives, ignorant of their state! One month later, the population of overweight American adults had zoomed to 97 million, or 55 percent of the adult U.S. population. No, it wasn't a bizarre experiment by a race of mate-hunting alien beings who find Paul Prudhomme the acme of sex appeal. The government did it, via the Body Mass Index (BMI) guidelines released by a seriously compromised task force of the National Institutes of Health. (One of the most serious compromises of its integrity was the involvement of the FDA's Michael Weintraub in the writing of the guidelines: Weintraub was the leading academic promoter of the nightmarish diet drug fen-phen.)

The BMI has gradually replaced the 1959 Metropolitan Life Insurance Co. height-weight chart as the nation's leading (waistline) inflation index. The Body Mass Index is one of those ridiculously complicated and not terribly meaningful statistics, like the NFL quarterback ratings or a baseball player's slugging percentage, that seems to have been devised by mathematicians with too much time on their hands and too many empty beer bottles on their table. To find your BMI—bet you didn't even know you had one—multiply your weight in pounds times 703. Divide the total by your height in inches squared. And there you are. Most of us fall somewhere between the low 20s and the middle 30s.

In the lax and liberal days of yore, the NIH relegated men with a BMI over 27.8 and women with a BMI of 27.3 or higher to the overweight category. But that was before obesity became a *disease*, and its cure a matter of national priority. Under the new regime of Thinness Über Alles, a BMI of 25 to 29.9 characterizes an officially overweight person. Those with BMIs of 30 and above are obese. You don't have to be Rosie O'Donnell or Dom DeLuise to hit the magical number of 30. A strapping jock of, say, 6'1" and 225-pounds is "obese," which means he runs a "high" health risk. Of what, you ask? The government will have to get back to you on that. But in the meantime, our 6'1", 225-pound athlete is a candidate for diet drugs, according to the federal guidelines.

If you joined the ranks of the newly fat, take heart: you're in fit company. Arnold Schwarzenegger scores a 27.7. Only two players on the entire 1998 roster of the Washington Redksins were not fat. (Good luck to whichever bureaucrat tells them to their faces.) Now, admittedly, some of the hulks in the National Football League are fat by any standard. Defensive lineman Dana Stubblefield, a 315 pounder, charts at 40.53 on the BMI, while 326-pound teammate Tre Johnson leads the Redskins at 41.94. But it is at what everyone but linemen call the "skill" positions that the BMI turns laughable. Cornerback Darrell

Table 3.1 Body Mass Index (BMI) by Height and Weight

Weight	100	110	120	130	140	150	160	170	180	190	200	210	220	230	240	250
Height																
5'0"	20	21	23	25	27	29	31	33	35	37	39	41	43	45	47	49
5'1"	19	21	23	25	26	28	30	32	34	36	38	40	42	43	45	47
5'2"	18	20	22	24	26	27	29	31	33	35	37	38	40	42	44	46
5'3"	18	19	21	23	25	27	28	30	32	34	35	37	39	41	43	44
5'4"	17	19	21	22	24	26	27	29	31	33	34	36	38	39	41	43
5'5"	17	18	20	22	23	25	27	28	30	32	33	35	37	38	40	42
5'6"	16	18	19	21	23	24	26	27	29	31	32	34	36	37	39	40
5'7"	16	17	19	20	22	23	25	27	28	30	31	33	34	36	38	39
5'8"	15	17	18	20	21	23	24	26	27	29	30	32	33	35	36	38
5'9"	15	16	18	19	21	22	24	25	27	28	30	31	32	34	35	37
5'10"	14	16	17	19	20	22	23	24	26	27	29	30	32	33	34	36
5'11"	14	15	17	18	20	21	22	24	25	26	28	29	31	32	33	35
6'0"	14	15	16	18	19	20	22	23	24	26	27	28	30	31	33	34
6'1"	13	15	16	17	18	20	21	22	24	25	26	28	29	30	32	33
6'2"	13	14	15	17	18	19	21	22	23	24	26	27	28	30	31	32
6'3"	12	14	15	16	17	19	20	21	22	24	25	26	27	29	30	31
6'4"	12	13	15	16	17	18	19	21	22	23	24	26	27	28	29	30

BMI	Health Risk Based Solely on BMI	Risk Ajusted for Comorbid Conditions or Risk Factors
19-24	Minimal	Low
25-26	Low	Moderate
27-29	Moderate	High
30-34	High	Very High
35-39	Very High	Extremely High
40+	Extremely High	Extremely High

Source: **http://www.drkoop.com**

Green, renowned as one of the fastest and most athletic players in the league, rates a 28.4. The fleet running back Terry Allen scored a 27.59. (These chubbos could finish a 100-yard dash while your typical 23 BMI was still at the 40-yard line.) Quarterback Trent Green was fat at 26.93—the exact same BMI as quarterback Jeff Hostetler, who from a fan's eye view looks like Abraham Lincoln on the football field. Other newly tubby athletes included Baltimore Orioles shortstop Cal Ripkin (whose 28 BMI would seem to warrant a nickname change from Iron Man to Donut Man), Ripken's all-star teammate Brady Anderson (27), and even Olympic gold-medal skier Picabo Street (25).

The doctor behind the BMI scare was Dr. Xavier Pi-Sunyer, with a name out of a lurid 1950s sci-fi thriller and a style to match. Unlike Dr. Koop, Dr. Pi-Sunyer passes at least one hypocrisy test. When the guidelines were released, he carried 168 pounds on his six-foot frame. For those readers who are not idiot savants with a flair for multiplying things by 703, or for those who haven't a calculator nearby, that translates to a BMI of 23.

Dr. Pi-Sunyer is a Barcelona, Spain-born obesity researcher and chairman of the National Heart, Lung and Blood Institute task force of the National Institutes of Health. He is also, signally, on the board of the American Obesity Association. "We felt that the record was clear and the risk was there,"[106] he said somewhat unclearly upon the release of the report.

"[T]he task force found that there is a higher risk for illness beginning at a BMI of 25,"[107] claimed Dr. Pi-Sunyer. He went on to say, "People can add a significant number of years to their lives if their BMI remains under 25." Well, not quite. This whopper, apparently grounded in the C. Everett Koop school of Unsubstantiated Assertion, was too much even for the infamous Judith S. Stern, vice president of the American Obesity Association. "The rationale behind these definitions is based on . . . data that shows [*sic*] increases in mortality with a BMI of 25 and above," said Stern. "They have misquoted the data. . . . if they are going to do it scientifically, they should do it scientifically. I would not change public health policy on that."[108] Stern was the lone dissenting vote on the NIH advisory panel. On the other hand, the *AOA Report* announced that "the risk of dying increases with each additional step in BMI, starting with a BMI of 25."[109] So there is one standard of truth for elite panels and another for the mere reader. The AOA did not bother to list the problems associated with *low* BMI, among them osteoporosis, athletic amenorrhea (loss of estrogen secretion, which leads to the stoppage of menstruation), stress fractures, low blood pressure, and sudden stopping of the heart (due to a lack of lean tissue or mineral deficiencies).

A.G. Britten, editor of *Mode*, a magazine for women who regard Kate Moss as a contemptible little twig, feared that the BMI guidelines "will put more than a few people into a much bigger panic about losing weight." Donna Britt in the *Washington Post* speculated that it would "increase the use of diet drugs."[110] Which indeed it will. Judith Stern explained her vote against Dr. Pi-Sunyer's brainchild as being motivated in part by fear of a "slippery slope. If the guidelines go out the way they are, there will be a big push to lower the BMI at which we treat with drugs and that's not justified, given the current drugs."[111]

Dr. Pi-Sunyer's response to criticisms of that sort was not quite a ringing denunciation of the diet drug racket. "Could more doctors turn to drugs?" asked Pi-Sunyer rhetorically. "That's a possibility. But we make it very clear in the guidelines that drugs should not be used by people who don't fit the criteria set by the FDA." In other words, place your faith in the sages of the Food and Drug Administration, the regulation-mad agency with a soft spot for diet drugs and a stance of deference to C. Everett Koop and the health police.

"We certainly have imperfect knowledge and therefore imperfect therapy" for weight control, conceded Pi-Sunyer. "But to say that people can't lose weight or at least maintain weight is being defeatist. We have evidence that people can do that. Look at all the lifetime members of Weight Watchers."[112] Yes, look at them: it is not defeatist but honest to say that there is no evidence that they maintain their initial weight loss. (Admittedly, those non-defeatists who reached for Redux lost poundage and kept it off unto the grave.)

When ABC.NEWS.com had Dr. Pi-Sunyer as a guest in the aftermath of the BMI report, some of those posing questions had the hint of panic in their cybervoices. One fellow said he was 5'8" and weighed 165 pounds; his BMI was 25. Overweight! Should he shoot for 24?

Most doctors would tell the poor fellow to relax: his measurements are well within range of the healthy. They would say, like Dr. John Foreyt, "I always tell my patients, 'Get a life.' Focus on healthy eating and more physical activity. Don't worry about your weight so much."[113] But not our Pi-Sunyer. "By losing 5 pounds and going from 25 to 24, you definitely decrease health risk,"[114] he told the man, who probably launched into a vain and expensive regimen of fitness clinics, if not diet drugs, in an attempt to lose those five measly pounds. (In moments of candor, even hirelings of the diet industry admitted that BMI was a shot in the dark. Dr. Ted Cicero of the Washington University School of Medicine, a consultant for pharmaceutical firms Interneuron and Wyeth-Ayerst, told an FDA committee that "for the most part this [BMI] is quite an arbitrary number . . . one could argue that 24 or 25 is just as reasonable as 27, 28, or 29."[115])

Richard Klein, a professor of French at Cornell and author of the mischievously witty *Eat Fat*, argues that the BMI "guidelines have the effect of justifying radical diets and other weight-loss measures, which in the long run promote obesity." They also lay the groundwork for oppressive new laws and regulations—for our own good, naturally. By defining more than half of adult Americans as officially fat, Washington has served notice that we are a corpulent, slothful people, unable to take care of ourselves. We need the benevolent guidance of the Wise Men of Washington. "Our worst fears lead us to perceive in these harsher guidelines incipient forms of government coercion over our most intimate choices," writes Klein. "[U]nder the guise of giving us helpful suggestions, the government is setting new norms against which our failures of self-care will henceforth be measured, disapproved, and eventually punished."[116] When bon-bons are outlawed, only outlaws will have bon-bons.

Glenn A. Gaesser objected that "Aside from extremes, weight itself is irrelevant to health."[117] Also protesting the new standards were FDA officials from its Division of Metabolic and Endocrine Drug Products, who feared the guidelines "could create the erroneous impression that being overweight is a disease"[118]—which is exactly the point!

Believe it or not—*mirable dictu*!—one of the sharpest critics of the new BMI guidelines was . . . C. Everett Koop. "We have so many overweight and obese people in this country and we are trying desperately to get them down to weights that will be more protective," fretted Koop. "This makes it more complicated. I worry that people will say, 'This goes too far. I quit.' I think it is like someone being in a race and saying they moved the goal line."[119]

Eminently sensible, it would seem. As was Koop's charge that the new BMI guidelines "will confuse the public and the medical community. It needlessly stigmatizes millions of Americans and lacks a solid scientific rationale."[120] (For Koop to make that last assertion was on the order of astrologer Jeanne Dixon indicting the mind-readers of the Psychic Friends Network for superstition.) So was America's doctor changing his tune? Was he defecting from the hair-shirt side? No. He soon began repeating, "Knowing your BMI is just as critical as knowing your cholesterol count and blood pressure."[121] And Shape Up America! was signing on to the Partnership for Healthy Weight Management, which defined healthy weight as having a BMI of between 19 and 25. A man who is 5'10" and weighs just 130 pounds is a 19—he is healthier than Cal Ripken, or so says SUA!.

The AOA latched onto the BMI guidelines like an ambulance chaser gloms onto a little old lady who hurts her neck in a fender-bender. At the joint SUA!-AOA press conference to release the Wyeth-Ayerst-financed "Guidance for Treatment of Adult Obesity," President Richard Atkinson emphasized, "a BMI of 27 to 29, your risk of having a heart attack is doubled. Your risk of having cancer is doubled, the risk of having diabetes increases fourfold."[122] Standing by the good doctor as he spun his tale of horror was C. Everett Koop, whose BMI is 27.6. But then the rules don't apply to some people.

Koop, Stern, Atkinson, Pi-Sunyer: like frantic goldfish in a little plastic bag, the fat-fighters keep bumping into one another. For instance, Dr. Pi-Sunyer's work can be found under the imprint of Glaxo Wellcome, the pharmaceutical giant for which Dr. Koop did his well-compensated lobbying on patent issues. Glaxo Wellcome produces a journal, *Odyssey*, which it terms the "journal of innovation in healthcare." In August 1998 it published Dr. Pi-Sunyer's paper "Obesity research and clinical management," which begins with a lament that "100 million people [around the world] now have a body mass index greater than 30." Where is famine when you really need it? From one side of the globe to other, "more people are overeating" than ever before. After assessing the possible genetic causes of obesity, and the dangers of overweight (lower rates of suicide aside), Pi-Sunyer gets down to solutions. And given that Glaxo Wellcome sponsors *Odyssey*, is it any surprise that this American Obesity Association advisor sees the greatest hope for combating obesity to lie in "long-term . . . drug therapy"? He praises the work of Dr. Michael Weintraub, best known for his seminal work on fen-phen, and in fact Pi-Sunyer judges fen-phen to be "modestly effective in improving the possibility of weight loss." Not a word slips about its lethal side effects, but then perhaps the paper was composed before the FDA's recall. You know how poky those academic journals can be.

Dr. Pi-Sunyer concludes on a note of sunny optimism, reminiscent of those Dow Chemical commercials in which flowers bloom and birds sing, all because the technologists are at work. "Pharmaceutical companies have large teams at work in an effort to develop new medicines, and it is likely that more powerful drugs will be marketed in the future."[123] Undeniably true, and no one is more respectful than the authors of the combination of genius and perseverance that it takes to develop an effective and life-saving drug, but there is just something so . . . smarmy . . . about the whole Koop-Atkinson-Pi-Sunyer crowd and the appearance it gives of researchers for hire. Science deserves better.

4

Fen-Phen and the Koop Coup

"If they recommend 'no', these doctors ought to be shot."[1]

—Dr. Judith Stern, American Obesity Association on the FDA's vote to approve the sale of dexflenfluramine

With fen-phen and Redux, the killer diet drugs of the 1990s, all our old friends come together: C. Everett Koop, Dr. Richard Atkinson, leading his one-member advocacy organization for 70 million people, the irrepressible Dr. Xavier Pi-Sunyer, and the stern Dr. Judith Stern, would-be organizer of the first firing squad in FDA history.

Fen-phen was the pharmacological application of the schoolboy belief that if you place one foot in a tub of ice and the other foot on a bed of hot coals, you've achieved climactic equilibrium.

The first, phonetical fen is short for fenfluramine, which depresses the appetite by increasing the activity of serotonin, which makes the patient feel full. Dope up Dom DeLuise with the stuff and he'd push away from the table with a half a plate of foie de gras left. The second phen is shorthand for the amphetamine phentermine.

Fenfluramine, which was approved by the FDA in 1973 for use as a controlled substance, was marketed under the name Pondimin; phentermine is most commonly denominated Adipex-P, Ionamin, or Fastin. The drugs had been legal for years but were no great shakes on the diet-pill market, for the side effects were nasty. But then along came University of Rochester pharmacological researcher Michael Weintraub, who later was to work for the FDA. In 1992, Weintraub had a brainstorm, rather in the way that some enterprising primitive first slathered peanut butter with jelly, or mixed oil with vinegar, or combined sour mash with a hemp cigarette. What if the side effects of fen nullified those of phen; and vice versa? Cross sleepiness with sleeplessness and what do you get? A skinny client and a fat bank account.

Weintraub's sample included 121 patients, two-thirds of them women, with an average weight of 200 pounds. Those who combined an exercise regimen with a daily doping of fen-phen lost, on average, 16 percent of their body weights (or thirty pounds) over eight months; those taking a placebo along with exercise lost an average of five percent of their body weights, or ten pounds. What desperate dieters did *not* learn from the fen-phen hype is that nineteen subjects of the Weintraub study dropped out, bothered by severe side effects, and that "*[n]one of the dieters maintained the weight loss after going off the drugs*."[2]

Weintraub's study, funded by the National Heart, Lung and Blood Institute (i.e., you) and published in the May 1992 issue of *Clinical Pharmacology and Therapeutics*, was widely reported in such venues as the *Washington Post*. "When people hit the wall with nonmedication interventions, where it becomes increasingly difficult to lose weight and people become discouraged, then medications can play a role,"[3] he said. Not a supporting role, mind you, but one worthy of Marlon Brando at his most expansively hammy. (Weintraub later said he had a difficult time finding a publisher for his study: "Journals were loath to print articles extolling the benefits of drug therapy. And it looks like they were right."[4])

Other studies followed. The ubiquitous Dr. Richard Atkinson of the American Obesity Association announced a five-year examination of fen-phen; not surprisingly, his early findings showed "dramatic weight loss"[5]—but then his subjects were simultaneously put on a 1,200 calories-a-day diet and given weight-loss counseling. Who wouldn't lose weight, at least for the short term? The drugs seemed to "change the chemistry of an obese person more toward the chemistry of a lean person," observed Atkinson, who believed that the bad old days—when "anyone who used obesity drugs was a little suspect"[6]—were gone for good.

Prescriptions of fenfluramine shot through the pharmacy roof after Weintraub's claims were publicized, rising from a mere 39,000 in 1991 to 65,000 in 1992, 155,000 in 1993, 282,000 in 1994, and then upwards of a million by the next year. Pharmacists were unable to keep the stuff in stock, even though the production lines at Wyeth-Ayerst were running 24 hours a day. "[W]e're in a back-order situation,"[7] said Wyeth-Ayerst spokeswoman Audrey Ashby, happily.

The drugs seemed to work; Dr. Steven Lamm, a Manhattan internist who treated hundreds of patients with the combination, wrote that his average patient lost six to twelve pounds in the first month and three to five pounds per month thereafter. Like most fen-phen prophets, Lamm took pains to emphasize that the combo was only for those in extreme circumstances—which in his case meant anyone with a BMI of 28 or more.[8] Everyone with a spare tire soon seemed to be on fen-phen. According to Dr. Charles L. Brown, medical consultant to the New Orleans Saints of the National Football League—and what kind of football team would hire a Charlie Brown?—many of the Saints were on the magic duo. Which might explain a few things about the perennially hapless Saints.

At first, the only obvious side effect was dry mouth. "You can be around food and you just don't have the desire to eat it," exulted fen-phen user Andrea Wagner to *Health*. "You don't even think about food."[9]

But what if there was a drug that killed the appetite like fenfluramine but didn't need the corrective stimulus of phentermine? Enter dexfenfluramine.

Dexfenfluramine, or Redux, needs no partner in combination. It releases serotonin into the brain, which increases "satiety"; that is, it makes the subject, human or animal, fuller faster. It also "suppresses the inappropriate craving for carbohydrates," in the somewhat odd formulation of one hired gun for Redux. This "inappropriate craving"—Nabokov's professor had one for pubescent girls, others of us have it for Twinkies—"drives a lot of people to overeat snacks, snacks which unfortunately are also full of fat which can contribute many calories."[10] So by stifling the constant craving for carbos and making the guinea pig feel as though his gut is going to bust after a couple of pretzels, dexfenfluramine reduces calorie intake in human subjects by about 400–600 calories a day.

Dexfenfluramine is "basically just the fen molecule with a section lopped off that causes profound drowsiness (thus making phentermine's buzz unnecessary)."[11] It is the d-isomer of fenfluramine. And it was needed, so its supporters said, because human beings are no longer capable of regulating their own behavior. "We've got too much food," explained Redux advocate Dr. Charles Lucas of Royal Oak, Michigan. "We've got too much money to spend on food. . . . The brain has been set for leaner times."[12] So only by giving the brain incorrect signals—such as, "You're full" even though the body which the brain surmounts has eaten a small portion—can Americans lose weight. Fecund land, productive farms, cheap food, mouth-watering dishes: the evils of the modern world make for a long, long list.

It is hardly a magic bullet: about half of the subjects in long-term dexfenfluramine trials dropped out, and the rebound effect took over, as their weight ballooned and eventually exceeded their pre-treatment weight. But those who took the drug did experience modest weight loss: Dr. Leo Lutwak of the Food and Drug Administration's Division of Metabolism and Endocrine Drug Products noted that in controlled studies, those taking dexfenfluramine and adhering to an exercise and diet modification plan lost an average of 10 percent of their body weight, while those on just the exercise and diet plan lost from five to 7 percent of their body weight: a small but not insignificant difference. "[W]e can conclude," said Lutwak, "that dexfenfluramine appears to have a modest effect in promoting weight loss over the period of a year."[13]

Wyeth-Ayerst, on the other hand, was promising the moon: it boasted of one study in which two-thirds of subjects lost at least five percent of body fat and more than one-fifth lost upwards of 15 percent of their body fat.

Wyeth-Ayerst, it seems, had hit the diet drug jackpot. The company (parent: American Home Products) marketed Redux, which was manufactured by Interneuron Pharmaceuticals of Lexington, Massachusetts. (The Minutemen fought for *this*?) First-year sales of Redux were projected to exceed $600 million; it was "the first in a new generation of smarter, more promising anti-obesity drugs,"[14] gushed *Barron's* a bit prematurely. Redux cost less than $3 a day: a bargain if it worked, and a windfall at first for Interneuron, whose stock skyrocketed from $14 to $33 after Redux was cleared by the FDA. Biotech analyst David Crossen predicted that sales could soon reach $1 billion annually—a prediction that turned out to off by only, oh, a billion dollars or so.

But in 1996, the future was dazzlingly bright for those with a piece of Redux. And for Wyeth-Ayerst, that wasn't all: it had acquired A.H. Robins in 1989, and with it Pondimin (fen). Just in time for the fen-phen frenzy.

Covering all the bases, at about this time Wyeth-Ayerst was giving Shape Up America! and the American Obesity Association an unrestricted $100,000 grant to publish their "Guidance for the Treatment of Adult Obesity." It came as something less than a shock that the SUA/AOA guidelines, unveiled by Dr. Koop at a press conference, recommended these drugs as "useful."[15]

These were not niche drugs, last resorts for the grossly obese. The Redux label recommended that its use be restricted to persons with a BMI of 30 or greater (say, someone who is 5'10" and weighs 210 pounds) or those with a BMI of 27 or greater (5'10" and 185 pounds) in persons with diabetes or hypertension. In other words, half the country might be popping Redux.

These drugs would be used in perpetuity, or at least until the taker met his or her maker. "I thought it was silly to treat a chronic disease with drugs for only short periods of time,"[16] said Dr. Louis Lasagna, a hired gun for Interneuron. If you wish to be thin for life, you've got to get hooked for life.

There was just one hurdle: the Food and Drug Administration. Created in 1928 as the Food, Drug and Insecticide Administration, it soon shed the bugs but otherwise steadily expanded its bailiwick until it took in "everything in our food supply except meat and poultry, all prescription and nonprescription drugs, cosmetics, breast implants, the nation's blood supply and prescription drugs used to treat animals."[17] The agency is a bastion of nannyism: one minute it is overseeing claims on restaurant menus, the next it is denying admission to the U.S. market of drugs used to treat AIDS patients in foreign lands. Sure, they may be condemned to death without these unapproved medicines, but it's for their own good. Better dead than beset by annoying side effects.

And yet the FDA is like so many of the alphabet-soup agencies that dapple the Potomac landscape. When not hostile to private enterprise, it doles out favored treatment to those private (often quasi-private) enterprises that hire the costliest lobbyists or the shrewdest K Street legal sharks. Sometimes a nanny, sometimes a corporate lackey: such is the ambiguous position of the Food and Drug Administration. Corruption, even bribery (or bribery masquerading under a Washingtonian euphemism) are the consequences of granting such virtually limitless powers to an agency of unelected bureaucrats, insulated from the effects of their actions (such as the untold number of deaths resulting from the glacial pace of drug approval and the incalculable cost of the FDA's ingrained bias against unconventional treatments).

The FDA was on display in all its inglorious contradictions on three autumn days in 1995. C. Everett Koop and the diet-drug behemoths came a calling to the open sessions of the Food and Drug Administration's Endocrinologic and Metabolic Drugs Advisory Committee meetings. The topics: the approval of dexfenfluramine hydrochloride—Redux—and the removal of fenfluramine from the regulatory tentacles of the Controlled Substances Act. The first two meetings (September 28th on Redux and 29th on fenfluramine) were at the Parklawn Conference Center in Rockville, Maryland; the third was held in the Plaza Ballroom of the Holiday Inn Silver Spring in Silver Spring, Maryland. Henry G. Bone III, an apt name for an M.D., presided, but the presiding spirit was that of C. Everett Koop, M.D. and his creed: Big Brother for you, Big Profits for me.

In fact, the imposing Chick himself was there on September 28th, unofficially. He was not listed among the presenters, but the very first witness, Dr. Barbara Hansen, president of the American Society of Clinical Nutrition, began her remarks by noting that "I accidentally wandered into the wrong conference room today, and ended up down the hall talking with C. Everett Koop. And he was talking about his Shape Up America! program."[18] What the hell was C. Everett Koop doing at the Parklawn Conference Center? Did he really just *happen* to be there? This is a fairly striking piece of circumstantial evidence, along the lines of someone in Dallas on November 22, 1963 saying, "Oh, I was walking around Dealey Plaza and I just happened to see Sam Giancana." Very interesting indeed. (Also among those unofficially present was former Secretary of State Alexander Haig, best remembered, if not loved, for declaring "I'm in charge" after his president, Ronald Reagan, was shot by John Hinckley. Haig owned 200,000 shares of stock in Interneuron. The Secretary glad-handed members of the FDA advisory committee, presumably with the same soft touch that made him so reviled a figure within the Nixon and Reagan administrations he served.)

Hansen proceeded to address the conferees in Koop-speak. Obesity was "a disease that cannot be satisfactorily addressed by behavioral means."[19] So much for exercise and watching what you eat: if it is a disease, it can only be controlled by medicine. Such as Redux, for instance. Sure, "[w]e always must be concerned with safety," but "we must compare it to the extraordinary increase in health risk and morbidity that obesity carries."[20] The disease is a killer. Therefore, a lax approval policy is appropriate. Quite true—if indeed obesity is a disease. And yet the FDA has not applied Hansen's reasoning to the numerous other risk-fraught drugs it has summarily rejected or buried for years.

Hansen was but a warm-up for the inimitable Dr. Judith Stern of the American Obesity Association. Speakers at FDA hearings are required to list their conflicts of interest, but in the interests of brevity, Stern condensed these, for a full accounting might have dragged the hearing into the next month. "I am on the Advisory Board of a major weight loss company," she confessed, "and we [the AOA] have received money from multiple drug companies."

"What company is that?" asked Dr. Bone, to which Stern replied, "Pardon me?"[21] in the classic manner of the found-out child stalling for time, for her interlocutor's memory lapse, for the sudden appearance of a meteor, whatever. But she hastily named a few, including Servier, the French pharmaceutical giant that had marketed Redux since 1985 in Europe, and Interneuron.

Having quickly disposed of the question of who was paying for the words that came from her mouth, Stern snapped off a few Koopisms—"we are literally in the midst of an obesity epidemic," "the ultimate goal of AOA is to change public perceptions so that this disease is given equal status to such diseases as diabetes and heart disease and cancer"—and then got down to business. Noting that "there have been no new drug therapies approved by FDA for treating obesity since 1973," Stern urged the Advisory Committee to give Redux the green light.

She concluded, much as in a religious ritual, with an invocation of the deity. "I didn't know that Dr. Koop was next door. [Who *did* know?] We could bring him in to read this quote that he read . . . in January," which was, "To our shame, we have done almost nothing about this major health threat. The Government, the medical community, the health insurance companies, no one has done much to encourage Americans to prevent the obesity that is costing us and killing us [himself excepted on both counts]. All too often we fail to regard obesity as the disease it really is."[22] So, in the name of Koop, approve this drug.

Dr. Glenn Cooper, president of Interneuron Pharmaceuticals, kicked off his testimony with Koop's factoid that 300,000 Americans die each year from obesity.[23] Given that dexfenfluramine had been marketed in sixty-five countries around the world and treated some 10 million patients, wasn't it time for the U.S. to join the parade? (The mythical figure of 300,000 obesity-related deaths proved tremendously useful to Dr. Koop's sugar daddies. Supporters of Redux "cited the figure at least seven times at FDA advisory panel hearings on the drug."[24])

Cooper then introduced the lead animals in his dog and pony show. And familiar names they were. The first of the trio of "internationally recognized experts in epidemiology and clinical treatment of obesity"[25] was Dr. Theodore Van Itallie of the Columbia University College of Physicians and Surgeons. The second was Dr. JoAnn Manson of Harvard Medical School, and the final name was Dr. George Bray of the Louisiana State University Medical Center in New Orleans; Dr. Bray's name also appears on the Advisory Council of the redoubtable American Obesity Association.

These three were a veritable Tinkers-to-Evers-to-Chance of obesity drug shilling. Van Itallie bemoaned the 300,000 dead each year from obesity and no doubt incurred the wrath of his Weight Watchers-paid colleagues by noting that conventional weight-loss programs are virtually useless, as clients "tend to regain most or all of the lost weight within a few years."[26] But "pharmaco-therapy" offers hope, right Dr. Manson?

How right you are, Ted. Dr. Manson led her auditors on a highly selective tour of BMI information, concluding that "even moderate overweight confers an increased risk"[27] of mortality. She in turn handed the baton to Dr. Bray of the American Obesity Association. To combat this "chronic disease," Dr. Bray envisioned an anti-obesity treatment that was similar to that for hypertension, "where a stepped approach using individualized drugs"[28] has been successful. Given the eventual deaths of diet-drug users from primary pulmonary hypertension, Dr. Bray's remarks have an air of ghoulish prescience.

Despite dexfenfluramine's resemblance to amphetamine, Interneuron's Ph.D.'d advocates went out of the way to emphasize the differences. After all, the word "amphetamine" has the ring of illegality; people get arrested for possessing the drug without a prescription. Amphetamines are one target of the holy drug war that the U.S. political establishment and its public-health adjunct prosecute with such vigor and ruthlessness; there is no more fervent drug warrior than C. Everett Koop, the man next door, whose only complaint about this liberty-destroying, treasury-depleting jihad is that it doesn't cast its net wide enough to include cigarettes today (and fatty foods tomorrow?).

The laboratory evidence introduced by dexfenfluramine's supporters seemed to promise nothing but blue skies and tightened belts. Dr. Robert Y. Moore adduced a study purporting to show that after ninety days of treatment, the concentration of dexfenfluramine in the brains of subjects was minimal. Moreover, animals administered high-dose dexfenfluramine exhibited no neural damage.[29]

Double-blind, placebo-controlled weight-loss trials at dosages of 15 milligrams resulted in statistically significant poundage reductions. (Higher doses were not "extensively studied"[30] and thus not recommended, even by the house scientists.) Dr. Richard J. Wurtman did concede his reliance on "short-term studies,"[31] which were perhaps not appropriate for a drug that was to be used long term, but you can't blame Wurtman for putting the best face on the drug: the MIT professor was a cofounder of Interneuron in 1985.

Yellow flags were acknowledged and just as quickly stashed under the seat. Dr. Bobby W. Sandage, Jr., primly admitted to receiving reports from "national adverse reaction centers in Europe," but dismissed these as inevitable when dealing with such a widely distributed drug. "As might be expected when treating 10 million patients," Dr. Sandage began in a way that minimized the import of what was to follow, "a number of sporadic, serious and adverse events in association with Dexfenfluramine treatment have been reported . . . a single serious adverse event, primary pulmonary hypertension, has emerged as a possible epidemiological signal."

"Although no cases of primary pulmonary hypertension were observed in the controlled clinical trials, a cluster of several cases were observed . . . after Dexfenfluramine was marketed in Europe."[32]

But, Sandage was quick to add, "We believe Dexfenfluramine represents a new effective therapy for the management of obesity with a highly favorable safety profile given the morbidity and mortality of obesity."[33] The qualifier is the key: if obesity is a disease that kills 300,000 people each year, isn't it worth the risk of killing a few hundred or so with primary pulmonary hypertension so as to prolong the lives of the others?

There are few illnesses more relentlessly lethal than primary pulmonary hypertension (PPH), a very rare disease that has a survival period of 2.8 years—shorter than AIDS or most forms of cancer. The first reported case was in Germany in 1891; it remained exceedingly rare until the widespread use of amphetamine-like diet drugs. A person with PPH experiences a huge increase in the blood pressure in her pulmonary artery, which carries blood from the right ventricle to the lungs. (About 70 percent of those with PPH are women.) The only real treatment is a risky lung transplant—and even if that takes, most recipients will die of transplant-rejection disease within a few years.

The job of finessing the teensy complication of primary pulmonary hypertension fell to Drs. Gerald A. Faich, Lucien Abenhaim, and Stuart Rich. Dr. Faich noted that in the 1960s, a diet drug called Aminorex induced an epidemic of primary pulmonary hypertension in Switzerland, Austria, and Germany.[34] A smaller, subsequent cluster led to an International Primary Pulmonary Hypertension Study (IPPHS), of which Dr. Abenhaim of McGill University in Montreal was the principal investigator. It should be noted—though few speakers bothered to do so—that the IPPHS was sponsored by Servier, which was marketing Redux in Europe. To the astonishment of only the terminally naive, the IPPHS found that there was really nothing to worry about.

The IPPHS located ninety-five cases of primary pulmonary hypertension. Of these ninety-five, 21 percent of the sufferers had been exposed to anti-obesity drugs. The investigators concluded that such medications were an independent risk factor for PPH, but Dr. Faich brushed this off as a virtual irrelevance. After all, he reasoned, "if obesity is one of the risk factors for primary pulmonary hypertension, it should be no surprise that a treatment will also be associated." No big deal. But it *is* a big deal: the treatment was an *independent* risk factor, by Faich's own admission. Which makes his next statement—that the relationship between certain anti-obesity drugs and PPH is "sort of the innocent bystander effect"[35]—particularly grotesque.

"There is no epidemic here," said Faich of the European cases of PPH. Besides, we must balance the "possible deaths induced by anti-obesity agents . . . against the potential benefits because we've been hearing a lot about the mortality consequences of obesity."[36] Three hundred thousand, three hundred thousand, three hundred thousand. . . .

Dr. Abenhaim conceded a link "between anorexigen use and PPH," since "people who had recent exposure had a higher odds ratio." After discontinuing the drug for more than a year, the odds ratio of contracting PPH dropped "to nonsignificant levels." The longer the use, he told the panel, the higher the odds ratio.[37] (Dr. Rich resisted the perhaps predictably politically correct effort of FDA committee member Nemat Borhani to include cigarette smoking among the risk factors for PPH. "[I]n all honesty," Rich told the no doubt crestfallen Borhani, "we cannot make the recommendation based on any scientific data that cigarette smoking is causative, contributory for, or aggravating PPH."[38] Not that "scientific data" underlie every other ascriptive evil of cigarette smoking.)

Two members of the PPH trio, Doctors Stuart Rich and Lucien Abenhaim, had links to Servier. Dr. Rich had served as a paid consultant to the company, which is why it was no shock to hear him downplay the "low susceptibility"[39] of human subjects to PPH. Dr. Abenheim received consulting fees from Servier for interpreting the International Primary Pulmonary Hypertension Study.

For the FDA, Dr. Leo Lutwak of the Division of Metabolism and Endocrine Drug Products insisted that the committee carefully consider the European cases of primary pulmonary hypertension traceable to dexfenfluramine. "In 40 years of medical practice, I've seen only one case," said Dr. Lutwak. "And it was frightening. It is a bad disease. And when I came across approximately 100 cases of primary pulmonary hypertension in association with the drug, this was frightening."

Most of these poor souls were women, noted Dr. Lutwak; their average BMI was about 31, with a range of 19 to 44. Many were taking both dexfenfluramine and fenfluramine: desperate, it seems, for the magic pill that would shed the avoirdupois. One disturbing feature of this unlucky hundred was that one-fifth "had BMIs that generally would be considered not warranting treatment with potent drugs."[40]

The dissenting voices that addressed the FDA committee came on after the Interneuron dog and pony show had finished to the rousing acclamation of at least one committee member. Dr. Nemat Borhani, professor emeritus at the University of California-Davis, gushed, boyishly, "This was a very comprehensive presentation. I thank you. It was beautiful."[41] Never had primary pulmonary hypertension been glossed over so prettily, with such style and panache. Dr. Borhani was a regular cheerleader for the Interneuron team. He greeted team captain Louis Lasagna as "my dear old teacher,"[42] which is not ordinarily the prelude to a grilling. But then lasagna is best when not grilled.

The dissenters had their say. Dr. Lewis Seiden of the University of Chicago interrupted the FDA-Interneuron love-fest with a powerful and meticulously documented examination of the neurotoxicity of fenfluramine in animals and humans. Beginning with a diffident "Well, let me see if I can disagree without being too disagreeable,"[43] Dr. Seiden demolished the case for fenfluramine and its cousin dexfenfluramine on both safety and efficacy grounds.

Dr. Seiden and his colleague, Dr. Mark Molliver of Johns Hopkins University, presented evidence of the damage that fenfluramine causes to brain serotonin neurons in animals—even after dosages are discontinued. The harm is irreversible. This effect is observed across the animal kingdom, from rats and guinea pigs to rhesus monkeys and baboons; the "logical inference," Seiden stated, "is that humans will be similarly affected."[44] Depleted serotonin levels in human beings produce "sudden severe depression or bursts of impulsive behavior."[45] The cure is worse than what ails you. But the cure, unlike the "disease" of obesity, was a potential gold mine. (And remember, fenfluramine clients are expected to take the drug over the long term; indeed, to their terminus.)

Dr. Molliver threw the committee for a loop with his un-disclaimer that "[w]e are not involved in clinical trials, preclinical trials, or production or sale of any particular drug."[46] Doesn't this boffin know how to make a buck? His slide show was not for the squeamish, featuring as it did rat brains, the cerebral cortex of a squirrel monkey, and other images that could make Teddy Roosevelt join PETA, all of which made the graphic case that fenfluramine leads to the swelling and then degeneration of serotonin axons in the brain. Such axons are regenerative—new ones grow in—but the "re-innervation isn't complete,"[47] Molliver pointed out. The regrowth doesn't quite reach the posterior regions of the cortex. The consequence of this "acute structural damage"[48] would be manifested, as Dr. Molliver says, in those characteristics related to serotonin: "mood, vigilance, and alertness."[49]

The long-term consequences of serotonin damage are unclear; besides mood swings, they may include "[loss of] memory function, sleep disorders, sexual function, impulsive behavior, and anxiety attacks."[50]

Dr. Borhani, he whose dear old teacher testified for dexfenfluramine, said that while all this talk of "neurotoxicity we heard today is very interesting and it is very informative . . . we are dealing with a very severe epidemic in this country, epidemic [*sic*] of obesity that is killing many, many thousands every year [at least he didn't say 300,000], and . . . I don't know whose fault it is [why does it have to be anyone's *fault*?], but for lack of a better suspect, I blame the . . . [drumroll, please] . . . pharmaceutical industries."[51]

The *pharmaceutical* industry? Yes, the pharmaceutical industry. It seems that not enough diet drugs were coming on the market: fenfluramine was approved in 1973 and no one took it until it became one-half of the fen-phen one-two punch. But rather than blame overly strict FDA regulation, for which a plausible case can be constructed, or the hype of the diet industry, Dr. Borhani, protector of the public weal, chastised the pharmaceutical industry—after which he urged the approval of dexfenfluramine, the product of that very same industry. Those heads in the room that were still awake after a grueling day of serotonin talk must have spun with wonderment. Summoning all the limited eloquence at his command, Dr. Borhani wailed, "I cannot live with my conscience tonight. We're dealing with a very severe epidemic of obesity with no medical treatment."[52] (One wonders how many consciences were vexed over the next two years, as the death toll mounted.)

Dr. Borhani was then one of only two committee members (out of eight polled) to respond in the affirmative to Chairman Bone's question, "Is the evidence of safety sufficient to warrant approval for long-term use as proposed?" (One other panelist later changed his vote to yes.) On the other hand, seven of the eight voted yes to the question, "Is the evidence of efficacy sufficient to warrant approval of dexfenfluramine for long-term indefinite use, as proposed?"

Thus they agreed with half of Dr. Seiden's contention that "the risks of fenfluramine are high [and] its potentials as a beneficial appetite suppressant are low."[53] Given the mixed vote, one might think that dexfenfluramine was laid to rest, at least for the nonce. Super-majorities of those advisory board members present and voting thought both (a) that it worked; and (b) that it was dangerous. But the matter did not lie there.

A second meeting of the Endocrinologic and Metabolic Drugs Advisory Committee was scheduled. This was "uncommon,"[54] panelists told the press. After all, the advisory committee had voted six to two (or five to three) that the potential harm caused by dexfenfluramine was sufficient to keep it off the market. A second chance was most unusual: it was as though a batter, after striking out in the World Series, was immediately given another at-bat—and this time, the defense didn't even have all its players on the field.

Meeting in the Plaza Ballroom of the Holiday Inn Silver Spring in suburban Maryland on November 16, 1995, that old gang was all there: Dr. Borhani, Barbara Moore, Judith Stern . . . but this time, there was no Dr. Koop skulking around in the next room. Instead, his eminence sent Barbara Moore to read a statement on his behalf. But what is equally interesting is who was *not* there: Doctors Seiden and Molliver, the leading scientific skeptics of dexfenfluramine, were in San Diego with other scholarly scourges of Redux at the annual convention of the Society for Neuroscience. Quite a coincidence, eh? The man most responsible for the holding of this highly unusual second-chance hearing, Dr. James M. Bilstad, Director of the FDA's Office of Drug Evaluation II, said, "Ideally, they [Seiden and Molliver] would have been there, but we didn't view [their absence] as a fatal lesion, by any means, in the process."[55] They were not, *pace* Dr. Stern, shot; they just weren't there.

Dr. Bilstad, that old smoothie, greeted the assembled at this second meeting with the bland claim that the earlier rejection of dexfenfluramine by the committee was based on a "misunderstanding"[56] of the question, which had appeared to be model of clarity to others who read it. He suggested that worries over PPH may have contributed to the no vote, but this disease was "a rare event."[57] More salient were the concerns over neurotoxicity raised by Doctors Seiden and Molliver, and what a shame it is indeed that these two men could not join us today. Oh well.

What we did not learn until later was that Interneuron had forwarded to the FDA a dossier attacking the anti-dexfenfluramine witnesses from the first meeting. Dr. Seiden was said to have given one-sided testimony (something Interneuron would never do); Molliver was accused of being friendly with scientists at Eli Lilly, an Interneuron rival. This cover letter to the dossier included this line from Interneuron president Dr. Glenn Cooper: "We appreciate Dr. [FDA Division of Metabolic and Endocrine Drug Products director Solomon] Sobel's decision that Drs. [FDA official Joseph] Contrera, Molliver, and Seiden all mentioned in the dossier will not make presentations on November 16th." Seiden, when apprised of the memo in 1998, said "I suspected something like this. I'm outraged. That's defamation of character." Molliver added, "The hearings are supposed to be discovery-type sessions. It seemed, by not having us there, they were attempting to silence any critics of the drugs."[58]

Among those addressing the committee at the November meeting were Lynn McAfee, the 500-pound representative from the Council on Size and Weight Discrimination. She was also a taker of fenfluramine, and while she testified that "there is no one in this room today who wants and needs this drug more than I do," presenting irrefutable visual evidence of her claim, she urged the committee to consider the fact that because "people gain back their weight once they stop taking anorectic agents, this is a drug one would have to be on for their entire lives."[59] Not a pleasing prospect, given the increased PPH risk for long-term users.

Over the course of the day the magnitude of that risk, and the risk of neurotoxicity, waned like a dying star. A succession of Interneuron—and Servier-subsidized researchers minimized the risks of this wonder drug. The dissembling started right off the bat, as Interneuron's Dr. Glenn Cooper blandly assured his listeners that "at the September 28th panel meeting, dexfenfluramine was neither approved nor turned down."[60] This is not true: it was turned down, but Dr. Bilstad's curious interpretation of the meeting was that panelists were so obviously confused, so inexplicably blinded to the merits of Interneuron's petition, that a mulligan was in order.

"[T]he Committee was [most] concerned about the issue of neurotoxicity,"[61] Dr. Cooper asserted, "[s]o we're going to be spending the lion's share of time today on that issue." He scoffed at "the complete lack of clinical significance of these high-dose animal toxicology studies."[62] Feed enough of any drug to an animal and you'll kill it. So what? And without Doctors Seiden and Molliver around to explain that modest doses had apparent neurotoxic effects, Cooper's remarks went virtually unchallenged.

"The drug has no abuse potential,"[63] Dr. Cooper assured the panel; a strange claim, since his minions had defended it against the neurotoxicity charge on the grounds that dosages were too small to worry about. Overdoses were another matter. Or perhaps he meant that unlike, say, marijuana, whose horrific side effects include a pleasant haziness and enhanced appetite, dexfenfluramine may send a few score consumers to grisly and rapid deaths but it does suppress the appetite—and isn't that what's important? In any event, Dr. Douglas Kramer of the FDA had elsewhere testified that high doses of fenfluramine (over 80 milligrams) were not uncommon; they produced "euphoria, hallucinations and other psychotropic effects." Sort of an LSD for mad dieters.

Panelist Dr. Robert Marcus objected to Cooper's claim, pointing out that "there's another epidemic," not of obesity but "maybe obesity standing on its head, and that is anorexia nervosa and other eating disorders" among young women "who are being encouraged all the time to get down below some arbitrary weight."[64] But Cooper soldiered on: "[t]he margin of safety for this drug is absolutely enormous."[65]

As for PPH, Dr. Taylor Thompson of Massachusetts General Hospital told the committee that almost half of those 101 European cases of dexfenfluramine-related primary pulmonary hypertension were either misdiagnosed or predated the victim's use of dexfenfluramine. Dr. Gerry Faich said that a central lesson of the International Primary Pulmonary Hypertension Study referenced earlier was that "dexfenfluramine and fenfluramine exposures of less than three months had little or no risk"[66]—but these drugs were intended to be used for life, not three months, so the relative harmlessness of extremely short-term exposure was meaningless. Faich also did a grim cost/benefit calculation, using Koop's inflated figures, and concluded that the risk to benefit ratio—lives saved by these drugs versus lives lost—was 144 to one.

The Koopian world was well-represented. The redoubtable Judith Stern, vice president of the American Obesity Association and urger-on of assassins of Redux skeptics, hit the usual series of low notes in succession—obesity is a disease, an epidemic, 300,000 will die this year alone—before giving the coveted AOA stamp of approval: "We strongly recommend that the development and approval of drugs to treat this disease be given special priority."[67] Given that her disclaimer credited Interneuron and Servier as sugar daddies, this is known as paying the piper. Stern dismissed neurotoxicity as irrelevant to human subjects and airily brushed away the "exceedingly small risk for developing primary pulmonary hypertension."[68]

Barbara Moore, executive director of Shape Up America!, read the statement of Dr. C. Everett Koop, who was perhaps lurking in other hallways, in other buildings, on this epochal day. Koop by proxy was at his Chicken Littlest. "The proportions of the obesity epidemic are enormous," he passed along, unpunningly. "It has already claimed one out of every three adults in the United States. It is seizing increasing numbers of children and young people, for whom the consequences will be most dire in terms of health care costs and human suffering. . . . The government should respond to this as a crisis. It should mobilize itself to address the problem on every front: in the home, in the community, in schools, and in the workplace. The FDA," he concluded, "can start the war today, by approving dexfenfluramine" and arming "every doctor's office across the United States."[69]

Warnings were scattered throughout the testimony; Dr. Paul Ernsberger, once a co-investigator on a $100,000 Servier research grant, stated, "If dexfenfluramine is approved by this Committee, it is certain that at least the minor epidemic of pulmonary hypertension will likely result."[70] Ho hum.

This time around, without the annoying clamor of dissenting voices, Interneuron prevailed. Some committee members did state reservations and objections: Dr. Robert S. Sherwin, noting the very short durations of most of the studies, suggested that "we may be underestimating the full presence of pulmonary hypertension over a relatively short period of observation."[71] Chairman Bone decried that "the neurocognitive testing that has been employed has been of rather poor quality at this stage." Moreover, he issued a warning: "We need to understand clearly that it's quite likely that if a million patients take this drug, at least a couple dozen of them will die annually as a result." Dr. Bone dismissed the cost-benefit calculations of Interneuron's hired guns as conjectures barely above the level of a guess. Moreover, "we have very little information about the actual reduction in mortality from weight-loss programs and, as far as I can see, no information at all about actual reduction in mortality from anorectic use."[72] So, the drug kills an unlucky few, and we don't really know that it saves any lives at all. Not surprisingly, Chairman Bone voted against dexfenfluramine.

But he couldn't carry his committee. On the key question of the day, "Based on currently available safety and efficacy data, overall benefits and risks in the use of dexfenfluramine, would you recommend approval for marketing?" the ayes were six and the nays were five. Formal final approval for the drug was granted on April 29, 1996, after which Redux was rushed to the nation's pharmacies by June. The standard daily dose was two 15-milligram capsules. The cost: a mere $2.40.

This is "a step in the right direction,"[73] proclaimed Dr. Xavier Pi-Sunyer.

Lost in all the fury over the two meetings to approve Redux was the September 29th joint meeting of the FDA's Drug Abuse Advisory Committee and the Endocrinologic and Metabolic Drugs Advisory Committee. The question was whether to remove fenfluramine and dexfenfluramine from under the Controlled Substances Act. The matter turned on the arcane question of the "abuse potential" of these drugs. The drugs were decontrolled; there was little discussion of PPH, as that had been covered at the previous day's contentious meeting.

The meeting was interesting only insofar as it provides even more evidence of the extent to which the Koopian health and fitness lobby is a virtual front for the pharmaceutical industry. Dr. Richard Atkinson of the AOA, who was at the time "the principal investigator on three separate studies"[74] concerning fen-phen—gosh, we wonder what he concluded?—told the panelists that dry mouth and constipation were about all that fen-phen users had to worry about. Dr. Ted Cicero, for Interneuron, urged the committee not to "forget [that] there are 290,000 deaths" each year "attributable to obesity"—a slight shaving of the nice round Koop figure. And for once, this number was challenged. Dr. Lutwak of the FDA, tiring of this pseudoscientific factoid, interjected, "That is a projection based on a hypothesis that has yet to be proven."

"I beg your pardon?" replied a nonplussed Cicero.

"I beg your pardon, sir," shot back Lutwak. "This is based on epidemiologic data which offer us the clue to where research has to be done. This is a projection. This is not 290,000 people dying off each year. . . . "[75]

* * *

By June 1996, Redux was selling for about $60 a month. Fen-phen went for $40 a month. The pills looked like the keys to the kingdom of wealth. The riches of Croesus beckoned.

On the *CNN Morning News*, no less an eminence than Dr. C. Everett Koop, while carefully disassociating himself from those who were overprescribing fen-phen and Redux as if they were going out of style—which, come to think of it, they were—urged these "very helpful" drugs for the "grossly and morbidly obese."[76]

Meanwhile, anti-Redux physicians were intimidated from voicing their reservations; as *Los Angeles Times* reporter Shari Roan wrote in October 1996, one doctor told her "that he fears legal repercussions if he says anything negative about the medication."[77]

The drugs had all the right endorsements. Recall from chapter 2 the estimable American Society of Bariatric Physicians, the dignified name that diet docs chose for themselves in a bid to swipe some prestige. The executive director of ASBP, James Merker, told the *New York Times* in February 1997, before all hell broke loose, that the Redux/fen-phen family "is very safe and effective provided it is being administered and closely supervised by a physician knowledgeable in the use of these medications."[78] In other words, by one of us. Mr. Merker turned out to be disastrously wrong, of course, but, hey: everyone makes mistakes, right?

Some physicians prescribed fen-phen as though it were Tylenol. Dr. Pietr Hitzig of Maryland boasted that he had 2,000 patients on the combination, which he called "a remarkable agent." Not only did they make fat people thin, they were "successful in stopping the addiction to alcohol, cocaine, heroin and other addicting substances"[79] and curing everything this side of the heartbreak of psoriasis.

Savvy doctors could tell which way the wind was blowing: they began to disparage conventional weight-loss programs and champion the wonder drugs.

Nutri/System was the first major diet center to incorporate fen-phen into its program, in 1995. The other lemmings were not far behind. Jenny Craig introduced Redux to its clients in late 1996; all 630 Jenny Craig centers soon had doctors ready, willing, and able to prescribe the pills. News of the drug's potentially fatal side effects did not quite come as a bolt out of the blue to the folks at Jenny Craig. In the company's fiscal year 1996 filing with the Securities and Exchange Commission, it admitted, "From time to time, medical and health professionals have identified health risks associated with weight loss. Weight loss pharmaceuticals, including dexfenfluramine, commonly referred to by its trade name Redux, while approved by the FDA, are not risk-free and side effects and potential health problems for certain users have been identified. Medical and scientific developments or public announcements associating a health risk with weight loss could have a material adverse effect on the Company."[80]

Well, that's one way of putting it. Though it must be conceded that the deaths of Redux and fen-phen swallowers had "material adverse effects" rather more severe on themselves and their families than on Jenny Craig—or Nutri/System, or any of the other weight-loss centers that promoted this panacea. "Weight loss medication is an effective part of the treatment of obesity, and if we are in the business of treating overweight people, we want to include everything available that works," said Joseph J. DiBartolomeo, vice president for scientific affairs at Nutri/System, in February 1997, speaking just a bit too soon. Responding to criticism by a Nutri/System doctor that the company was not testing the blood of potential pill poppers thoroughly enough, Dr. DiBartolomeo intoned, "What we learned was the medicines do work well and work very safely. That is the reason we stopped doing the blood work." Well, we can't all be Dr. Jonas Salk.

Nutri/System was especially dishonest on the matter of fen-phen. One of its brochures claimed that the study by Dr. Michael Weintraub of the University of Rochester found no harmful side effects after three and a half years of use. The brochure went on to make other claims of varying degrees of dubiousness, prompting Dr. Weintraub, usually regarded as the best academic friend fen-phen ever had, to protest that the Nutri/System's brochure "is not true to the spirit of the study. It is out of context, and I don't believe that is right."[81] To which the Hippocratic Dr. DiBartolomeo riposted that the brochure provides "the full picture." Nutri/System's practice was to prescribe fen-phen for up to two years, despite the general opinion, ranging from the *Physician's Desk Reference* to pharmaceutical-backed doctors, to limit use to three months. Of course the dieter who stopped at a mere three months soon would regain the lost weight and demand a refund or, even more chillingly, go across the street to Jenny Craig, so perhaps we ought not to be too hard on Nutri/System.

The typical diet-center doctor spent a whole ten minutes with a client before prescribing Redux or fen-phen. Dr. Israel Levavi, a physician toiling for one Los Angeles weight-loss clinic, told the *New York Times* that he examined six patients an hour in "very, very cursory exams."[82]

Morgan Downey of the AOA averred that "the vast majority of physicians only prescribed weight-control drugs for sound medical reasons, if they prescribed them at all."[83] Yet Dr. Robert Colton, a Florida-based diet researcher, spoke of doctors "giving this to people who just need to lose a few pounds, like a model."[84] There were tales of desperate dieters wearing hidden ankle weights so as to make a greater impression on the doctor's scale.

The Florida-based Advantage Weight Control was the first chain of clinics to hitch its star to fen-phen. The brainchild of a criminal lawyer and his wife—he really ought to have specialized in civil law, given subsequent events—Advantage charged $2,500 for a year-long regimen of visits with doctors, shrinks, counselors, and, most importantly, those little miracle pills. Far better, it turns out, to have spent the money on a year's worth of pizza and beer.

Never let it be said that we are stingy in giving credit when credit is due. Weight Watchers avoided Redux like a bowl of barbecued potato chips: "We're not a medical organization, and we never pretended to be. Medical decisions about prescription drugs should be left to people and their personal physicians,"[85] said spokeswoman Linda Webb Carilli. The group's Karen Miller-Kovach added, "I am worried that people are going to see this pill as a magic bullet. They are going to take this pill and sit on the couch and eat Haagen-Dazs and potato chips. And guess what? They are not going to lose weight."[86] Not quite true: Redux did work as an appetite suppressant. But nevertheless, Weight Watchers held out. So, there. Credit was given. In the spirit of generosity we shall refrain from dwelling on the point that Weight Watchers' relentless propaganda against the Devil Fat helped create the climate in which Redux might flourish. As Lynn McAfee, spokeswoman for the "fat acceptance" group, the Council on Size and Weight Discrimination, said in the midst of the fen-phen and Redux stampedes, "It has never been about these people [diet centers] caring about us. There will be financial incentives to keep people on these pills and that worries me a lot. These are serious drugs."[87] But then, what did Ms. McAfee know? After all, she was only another fat girl.

Then came the fall. On September 15, 1997, the FDA pulled dexfenfluramine (Redux) and fenfluramine (Pondimin) from the market; the other half of fen-phen, phentermine, remained on the market, but it was lost without its partner, rather like Sonny without Cher.

The withdrawal was not exactly a pious act of contrition. It took a three-hour meeting with FDA officials in Rockville, Maryland before Wyeth-Ayerst and Interneuron cried uncle and announced that Redux and Pondimin were history. Wyeth-Ayerst also took Pondimin off the shelves in Mexico, Canada, and Colombia; Servier followed suit in Europe. (The FDA's James Bilstad, the man who may have kept the anti-dexfenfluramine scientists from the second hearing, said, "I think our decision to approve Redux was justified at the time. It was approved based on the benefits and the risk."[88])

Till then, the FDA had only retracted a drug certified as safe three times in the previous decade. So this was not an ordinary occurrence, a typical bureaucratic snafu. The FDA's request that the manufacturers withdraw these products for the "unacceptable risk" of heart valve damage halted one of the most remarkable pharmaceutical stories of the age: In just over a year since its approval, two million Americans had taken Redux; four million had taken Pondimin since 1973, and the vast majority of those had done so since Michael Weintraub's seminal research was published in 1992. Between 1992 and 1997 more than 18 million prescriptions had been written for Redux and fen-phen.

The beginning of the end for the Redux revolution and the fen-phen fantasy had come in July 1997, when Mayo Clinic doctors reported severely damaged heart valves in twenty-four women who had taken fenfluramine or dexfenfluramine. Eventually, five medical centers examined 291 drug-taking dieters and reported that an astounding ninety-two had damaged heart valves. Under normal conditions, two or three would have been so afflicted. A study in the *New England Journal of Medicine* reported that up to a quarter of fen-phen users developed valvular heart disease. "This is one of the most serious incidents of drug injury that we've had in recent years,"[89] said Thomas J. Moore of George Washington University Medical Center.

Mayo Clinic Doctor Heidi Connolly did much of the sleuthing. Patient Number One exhibited heart-valve damage that could only be caused by one thing: the excretion of vast amounts of serotonin into the blood stream. When the patient confided, "I'm not big on taking pills, but I have been taking fen-phen for about two years,"[90] the jigsaw pieces began to fit. The serotonin irregularities predicted by the silenced duo of Drs. Seiden and Molliver had perhaps not been quite as irrelevant as Interneuron's flacks had claimed.

Typical of those suffering irreversible heart-valve damage from fen-phen was Sabine Sisk-Bisson of suburban Washington, who was no Lynn McAfee tipping the butcher scales at 500 pounds but rather an attractive middle-aged woman who wanted to lose the fifteen pounds she had gained since she quit smoking. Her doctor complied, and in 1995 she became an avid user of the drug cocktail. "I loved those pills," she reminisced three years later, after her first round of open-heart surgery. "You still looked forward to good food, but when it was put in front of you, you only wanted to take a few bites."[91]

Within months, she was having trouble breathing. Tests revealed an enlarged heart, and soon she was patient number four in the Mayo Clinic study that led to the withdrawal of fen-phen from the market. She was also among the first fen-phen victims to receive a settlement from American Home Products.

The Mayo Clinic reports seeped into the press; by late summer 1997, weekly prescriptions for Redux had dropped 52 percent from February; fenfluramine prescriptions had plummeted by 63 percent. "People are so fearful that they want no part of the drugs," said Robert Nierman, a Massachusetts diet-center surgeon who had promoted the magic bullets to his clients. "The decline is absolutely off the charts. We're fighting for survival now."[92] Analysts who had predicted $1 billion annual sales for Redux were revising estimates downward faster than their calculators could compute. Nutri/System frantically shifted clients from fen-phen to phen-Pro, the "Pro" being Prozac. A nation of artificially happy dieters was in the offing. But still, the desperate, whether model-envying teenage girls or overweight women frantic to avoid becoming one of Koop's 300,000 corpses, kept popping the pills.

Read enough of them and the Redux and fen-phen tragedies fit a numbing pattern. Mary J. Linnen of Quincy, Massachusetts, a hale and hearty tennis player, wanted to lose twenty pounds to fit into her wedding dress. She took fen-phen for twenty-four days; half a year later, she was dead of primary pulmonary hypertension. "Instead of walking down the aisle before a bride," her mother said, "I walked behind a casket."[93]

Using a Freedom of Information Act request, Kathleen Kerr of *Newsday* reported in October 1997 that between 1974 and 1997 the FDA had received at least seventy "adverse reaction" reports on fen-phen from doctors, pharmacists, and drug manufacturers—yet the agency, so ferocious in refusing approval to drugs that might actually save lives, took no action. Twenty-eight of these adverse reaction reports noted heart-related problems; fourteen suggested primary pulmonary hypertension. But the accumulating evidence was never weighed by an arbitrary and capricious bureaucracy. The most chilling response to the *Newsday* story came from Dr. Terrance Coyne, vice president of medical affairs for Medeva, the makers of a form of phentermine marketed as Ionimin. "A death," said Dr. Coyne in his best Strangelovian accent, "is not an adverse reaction. It's an event—an outcome."[94]

Taking the cake, so to speak, for the most shameless spinning of the fen-phen and Redux disasters was the American Obesity Association. Two months before the recall, its president had declared that all was well; the vice president had earlier said that FDA panelists who did not approve dexfefluramine should be shot. So was there a public apology, an act of contrition by the AOA? You gotta be kidding. Instead, the organization boasted in its promotional material, "The AOA issued two statements in the summer and fall of 1997 regarding the investigation and later recall of obesity drugs. Both statements received widespread media attention. The AOA has handled hundreds of press inquiries into obesity generated by the recall of fenfluramine and dexfenfluramine."[95]

So this is what it comes down to. After shamefully shilling for killer diet drugs, the AOA brags that it "received widespread media attention." Well, so did Charlie Manson! Seldom has the trickle-down effect of the cult of celebrity been so baldly displayed: it doesn't matter *why* one gets into the newspaper or, even better, on television, all that matters is being on TV! If they had even a smidgen of honor, Atkinson and Stern would have closed up shop after fen-phen and Redux dug their patients' graves. And C. Everett Koop would have resigned from the AOA Advisory Council. But that would be asking for decency—that would be asking, in other words, for too much.

Dr. Atkinson, in particular, ought to have burrowed underground for a decade or two as contrition. He had told the FDA's joint committee meeting of September 29, 1995 that of the 428 patients he currently had on weight-loss regimens, an astonishing 87 percent were taking either fenfluramine alone or the fen-phen combination.[96] This Dr. Feelgood makes Elvis's doctors look like Marcus Welbys.

Amusingly, when in the week after the September 1997 recall the *Los Angeles Times* convened a panel of "experts" to answer questions about the fiasco, Dr. Richard Atkinson was queried, "Which is better, to taper off or to quit these drugs cold turkey?" To which he replied, "I think it's better to taper off over a week or so"[97]—good to the last granule, it seems.

(At least one organization did not do a volte-face over the drugs: James F. Merkler, executive director of the American Society of Bariatric Physicians, said after the withdrawal, "Many of our physicians are rather skeptical and perplexed as to why nothing more than an observational report [i.e., ninety-two of 291 patients experiencing valve damage] would have such great weight."[98] This is the plaint of a man whose ship has just gone out.)

After the recall, Morgan Downey, the recovering fat person who is executive director of the AOA, went into a spin cycle worthy of Bill Clinton's most accomplished liars-for-hire. The group's earlier defenses of the drugs were soft-pedaled: "we were concerned by the Mayo Clinic findings," Downey claimed, "But we cautioned against overreaction." They were acting responsibly, as scientists and medical persons ought to, while all around them the flighty were losing their heads. But just as turf-seizing, power-hungry Washington pols are always doing it "for the children," the AOA is ever-concerned with protecting the fat. (Or the one person— fat or not, we don't know— who is a real live member.)

"Our first priority was to ensure that persons with obesity were not incurring serious heart valve damage or other health effects,"[99] Downey announced gravely. Apparently this priority was of recent vintage, postdating Dr. Stern's declaration that FDA panelists who hesitated to approve Redux ought to "be shot."

As for Dr. Koop, the mysterious man in the next room during the FDA hearings, he spun hard for his friends at the FDA. The regulators "conducted a lengthy and comprehensive review based on all the science that was currently available," he declared after his sugar daddies had withdrawn the drugs from the market. "The agency acted responsibly and consulted the leading obesity researchers and medical authorities before reaching its decision. Appropriate analysis of risks and benefits was conducted using the data at hand. There are no reasons for recriminations: FDA did its job and did it well." Above all, he thundered in best martial voice, "the war on obesity must continue unabated."[100]

After the deaths came the deluge. More than 1,000 lawsuits against American Home Products and Interneuron are at various stages in the courts, and the tea leaves look worse than bitter for the drug peddlers. In the first major decision, a Canton, Texas jury ordered American Home Products to pay $23.4 million to thirty-six-year-old fen-phen user Debbie Lovett, whose heart-valve damage was traced to Pondimin.

But the search for the magic pill goes on. Other companies designing appetite suppressants or purported fat-fighters include Knoll Pharmaceuticals, Roche Laboratories, Hoffmann-La Roche . . . the list is lengthy, many of the names familiar to those who read the financial statements of Shape Up America! and the American Obesity Association. As George Washington University Obesity Management Program medical director Arthur Frank says, "Every drug company in the world is working on developing diet drugs."[101]

As always, there are starts and fits, fires and misfires. One of the most promising drugs of recent years, Hoffmann-La Roche's Xenical, which blocks the absorption of fat in the intestinal tract, seemed to work in clinical trials, though with the unpleasant side effect of "loose stools that can cause soiled underwear." Frances Berg of *Healthy Weight Journal* notes that Xenical produces "Explosive diarrhea when you least expect it"[102]—not exactly a good date drug. It also seems to inhibit the absorption of Vitamin D and may be linked to breast cancer, but hey, isn't losing 10 percent of your body weight worth it?

Upon Xenical's approval by the FDA in the spring of 1999, analysts predicted annual sales of up to $1 billion. Sound familiar? A month's supply of the drug cost $100, and although it is recommended for those who BMIs are 30 or above, doctors can prescribe it to anyone—and if fen-phen and Redux are any guide, they will.

Dr. Frank, for one, does not believe that the disasters of fen-phen and Redux will scare off pill-popping dieters: "Instead of abandoning [pills] I think people are going to be more careful about using medications."[103] For instance, there has been no rush to use Meridia, one of the very few weight-loss drugs still on the market, which makes the user feel full after eating (it also boosts blood pressure and interacts badly with Prozac or Zoloft).

The race is also on to manipulate the obesity gene ob, discovered by researchers at Rockefeller University and sure to make the researchers, and Amgen, which shelled out $20 million for the commercial rights, as rich as Rockefellers—if, that is, the treatments for obesity based on ob and subsequently discovered "obesity genes" actually work, and are not simply biotech versions of fen-phen.

The next Big Thing will find a wary public and millions of potential users who know far more than they would like to about serotonin, valvular damage, and primary pulmonary hypertension. Doctors Koop, Atkinson, and Stern have their work cut out for them—but it's nothing that a million dollar grant here, a half-million dollar grant there, wouldn't make easier. Wyeth-Ayerst, open that checkbook.

5

Koop: The Brand Name

"I have never been bought," [Koop] said. "I cannot be bought. I am an icon, and I have a reputation for honesty and integrity, and let the chips fall where they may."
—*New York Times*, September 5, 1999

". . . drkoop.com should really be named drkoop.con . . . [or perhaps] drkook.com."
—Steve Milloy, Junkscience.com, September 29, 1999

"I think people believe me," said Dr. Koop in 1994. "That's why it's important that I'm the figurehead for this campaign."[1] Which campaign, you ask? It really doesn't matter. What counted was the cash, and C. Everett Koop was to find that when "people believe me," being a figurehead was a virtual key to the treasury.

C. Everett Koop has made retirement pay in a way that awes even jaded Beltway denizens. The typical ex-cabinet official takes a modest office in a closet or anteroom of a pricey D.C. lobbying firm and is hauled out when appropriate to shake a few hands and grease a skid or two. It's a sleazy business, but it's a living.

But not enough of a living for former Surgeon General Koop and the smoke-free Betty. He, after all, had breakfasted with Morgan Fairchild and made a documentary with the anorexic—no, sorry, the preternaturally slender—girl on *The Partridge Family*. His volubility on AIDS, after years of cowardly silence, had brought him into contact with what is pretentiously known as the Film Community, so it was only fitting that the good doctor chose for an agent the oily Norman Brokaw, Chairman and CEO of the William Morris Agency.

Brokaw started in the mail room with William Morris in 1943; being a "talent agent" is his life. His office is in Beverly Hills; among his clients are Brooke Shields, Priscilla Presley, and Gerald R. Ford, and if you can spot a talent in the bunch you have keener eyes than we do. (In fairness, he also represents Bill Cosby and Andy Griffith.)

Among the deals Brokaw brokered for Koop was his joining Mbf USA, Inc. (surely one of the murkiest and least-revealing corporate names) as chairman of its Advisory Board. Now, the advice these boards give is usually limited to, "Make more money," but in the case of Mbf USA, America's doctor brought a certain expertise. His job, as *Business Wire* reported, was to be "instrumental in guiding the Company's entry into the global vitamin supplement and nutritional product market."[2] Which dovetails nicely with his full-time occupation of America's nag, exhorting us to pay more attention to—nay, obsess about—our nutritional lives. The deficiencies therein, it would seem, can be corrected by a pill here, a pill there.

Ralph Waldo Emerson said that a foolish consistency is the hobgoblin of small minds, in which case Dr. Koop's mind is cavernous indeed. For in accepting his position with Mbf USA, which included his chairmanship of the nonprofit Mbf USA Foundation, Koop declared that combating *hunger* was a priority for him: "I believe our efforts could have a major impact on the eradication of hunger, which affects millions of Americans, and most dishearteningly, so many of them children,"[3] he oozed. Well, now. *Hunger* is the problem? We thought it was obesity! On one side of his mouth America's doctor tells us that we, his patients from sea to shining sea, are busting their belts in record numbers—especially children, and even babies, whose chubbiness we profess to find "cute" in our perverse way. Yet on the other side of his mouth Dr. Koop intones his concern that "millions" of us are hungry—especially children. We are, it seems, a nation of extremes: half of us gross and obese, the other half pathetic starvelings. But one man can save us, if only we give him the power and the glory (and a million-dollar contract). . . .

Mbf USA is about more than just pills (excuse us: nutrition supplements) and platitudinous sallies against hunger. Picking up on a favorite theme of the post-religious-right Koop, it proudly markets "the world famous Playboy (TM) brand condoms."[4] These, it should be said, do not bear the personal endorsement of Dr. Koop.

One product that does get Chick's personal endorsement is the redoubtable egg. In 1996, at the height of the cholesterol scare, the American Egg Board and the Egg Nutrition Center enlisted Koop as a pitchman for the much-maligned ovoid. Taking the high road, refusing to make the obvious puns on Chick and Koop and the products thereof, the ex-surgeon general touted the nutritional benefits of egg consumption and boasted that he ate these little cholesterol-packed spheroids every day.

Good for him: the anti-egg campaign was among the more foolish instances of dietary hysteria. But what on earth was Koop, the self-appointed four-star general of the anti-fat army, doing plumping for eggs? Was this part of a master scheme by which Koop would make money helping Americans put weight on and then catch them on the flip side, profiting as they popped pills and supplements to take the weight off?

Donald McNamara, executive director of the Egg Nutrition Center, said, "we require continued vigilance against the nutritional police. If you don't think they are out there, that would be a mistake."[5] Well, *of course* they're out there: their leader is on your payroll, for heaven's sake! (Or had McNamara been reading his Machiavelli when he signed Koop? Keep your friends close and your enemies closer and all that.)

Among the first corporate gravy trains Koop hopped aboard was BioPure Corp., a Boston biotechnology firm founded in 1984 to develop a blood substitute useful in transfusions. As Robert Pool wrote in *Science* magazine, modified hemoglobin would be a blessing on many counts: "Patients would not be exposed to the AIDS, hepatitis, and other viruses that sometimes lurk in donated blood; doctors would not have to worry about matching blood types; and blood substitutes could be stored longer and at lower costs than whole blood, which must be kept refrigerated and has a shelf life of only a few weeks."

There have been obstacles, to be sure, including kidney failure in the earliest human subjects. "It scared him so much that he got out of the field,"[6] said one colleague of Konrad Messmer, the Heidelberg University pioneer in blood substitute research.

But the rewards will be abundant to whichever company sets the pace in the field. BioPure was the early leader: in 1990, shortly after

C. Everett Koop joined the Boston group as chairman of its scientific advisory committee, BioPure sold rights to its as-yet undeveloped product to Upjohn for $25 million. The former surgeon general, priming the investment pump, predicts that blood substitutes "will rank in importance with antibiotics and the polio vaccine as one of the top ten medical advances of this century."[7]

The U.S. Army is among those most eagerly awaiting a blood substitute, for reasons that anyone who has ever seen an episode of M*A*S*H could detail. And wherever soldiers are found, C. Everett Koop is sure to be near. (Except in Arlington, much to the Surgeon General's chagrin. Though don't count him out even there just yet.)

Koop enraged Army doctors in 1990 when, after signing on to shill for BioPure, he lobbied Army officials to give a leg up to his corporate paymasters when it comes time to fill a medic's bag with modified hemoglobin. Koop earned his dollar: according to *Science*, "BioPure officials met . . . with the surgeons general of the various branches of the armed services to offer information about the company's blood substitute." One Army source told a journalist, "It's possible they [BioPure] have a good product, but they've been so goddamned secretive that they haven't allowed enough investigation of the product to generate a high level of confidence in the scientific community."[8] But then confidence is the game of C. Everett Koop, and whatever doubts mere Army doctors may have had about BioPure were trivial in comparison to the towering reputation of America's family doctor.

This is not particularly shocking: it's just the way the game is played in Washington, D.C. Companies purchase ex-officials of the federal government, who in turn provide the companies with access to those bureaucrats who know the combination to the federal exchequer. Big deal. Welcome to the real world.

But this is not how the "real world" of the American Republic was supposed to work, and given the sanctimonious pose struck by retiring Surgeon General Koop, he of the "integrity not for rent" shtick, this *is* a big deal. Or at least it is another brushstroke in the portrait of a phony.

As it turns out, BioPure is not quite ready for prime-time wars, not yet, though its blood substitute is used by vets—veterinarians, that is—on anemic dogs. Questions persist about its usefulness for human beings: the blood supply is safer than ever, and synthetic blood seems not to be a good match for those with high blood pressure. Its effect on the immune system is also problematic. Reading the blood on the wall, in 1996 Upjohn bought out of its agreement with BioPure—a serious blow to the company, but by then America's doctor had found even more lucrative sidelines in the integrity business.

Rent him by the year or rent him by the hour: Mr. Integrity aims to please. It got to be too much even for his new friends on the regulatory left: Ralph Nader's *Public Citizen* protested that the Koop Foundation had taken in a cool million from drug maker Schering-Plough and that Koop had helped extend Schering-Plough's patent on Claritin, its much-ballyhooed allergy drug. Yes, the doctor admitted, the foundation had taken in a million, and he had circulated a letter in April 1999 on behalf of legislation benefiting Claritin.[9] But he was Dr. C. Everett Koop: there was no connection whatsoever between the two events!

Some men take up woodworking or stamp collecting in their 70s and 80s; C. Everett Koop took up patents. When Glaxo, the British-owned pharmaceutical giant, put on a full-court press lobbying effort in 1995 to keep the Congress from reversing a legislative error that meant $3.6 billion for the company, it enlisted an array of lobbyists and economists and ex-senators and ex-Cabinet officers and rent-a-scholars and, marveled the *Journal of Commerce*, "even the saintly figure of retired Surgeon General C. Everett Koop." (Glaxo CEO Charles A. Sanders would later sit on the board of BioPure with C. Everett Koop. Small world.)

The issue was patent law, not theretofore known to be specialty of the sainted Koop, but hey, he's a fast learner. Glaxo's patent on Zantac, its popular anti-ulcer drug, was to expire, as patents do, but a mistake by the lawyers who drafted the patent-agreement language extended the Glaxo patent by 19 months. "No other patents were given such extensions," but if you think that Glaxo's lawyers said, "A mistake is a mistake; please redraft the language as it should be," then you would be as out of place on K Street as a Carmelite nun. Glaxo, while conceding that it was profiting by a drafting error, spent tens of millions of dollars pressing its case in Congress. Koop, as always seeking to pad his wallet while appearing as pure as the driven snow, spoke loftily of a "miracle drug" to ease "great suffering"[10]—which of course was magnificently beside the point. Senator Orrin Hatch (R-UT) continually adduced Dr. Koop in his arguments for giving Glaxo a break.

When his reputation took a hit in the press—the first bad copy he'd had since he was an evangelical right-to-life Reaganite, and how long ago those days seemed—he backed off and "expressed regret"[11] over his pro-Glaxo stance. He had been misled, he claimed. And he certainly was not a mere lobbyist. (Technically, this is true. Technically.) Glaxo CEO Robert A. Ingram wrote a groveling letter to the *Journal of Commerce* insisting that "To suggest that Dr. Koop's opinions could be bought maligns one of the most respected physicians in the country."[12] In the end, Glaxo won by a 49–48 vote in the Senate.

Regret notwithstanding, the Koop-Glaxo marriage endured. In September 1996, Glaxo Wellcome was the chief advertiser (27 pages) in a special edition of *Time* called "The Frontiers of Medicine." The lead essay was by Glaxo errand boy C. Everett Koop, who waxed technological about "information technology" slaking the "insatiable demand" of consumers for medical information. The Internet would "empower patients"[13]—in which case the doctor stood to make the riches of Croesus, as we will see. And as we shall also see, *Time* may as well have titled the issue "Flogging a Dead Horse," for its purpose was not to "empower" sickly readers but rather to sell the unsellable: the videotapes of the issue's star, the paladin of Glaxo, C. Everett Koop. In 1997, having long since gotten over his regret, the former Surgeon General was named to the advisory board of a Glaxo Wellcome-sponsored PBS series titled "Breakthrough: Television's Journal of Science and Medicine." Yes, Koop had spent the previous three years slamming TV for its role in flabbifying America, but by now he was such a thoroughgoing Pharisee that no one even bothered to keep track of the petty hypocrisies.

Koop had long received the kid-glove treatment from the media, but in late 1999 a handful of outlets gave him the latex-glove treatment. A *New York Times* editorial revealed that Mr. Integrity had made a 1997 phone call to Dr. Linda Rosenstock, director of the National Institute for Occupational Health and Safety, in which he told her that the agency's warnings about the dangers of certain latex gloves commonly used in hospitals were "way overstated." According to Susan Wilburn of the American Nurses Association, 17 percent of hospital workers with "heavy exposure" to the gloves have developed allergies, some quite severe.)

Two years later, Koop testified before a congressional House subcommittee that the latex gloves were a victim of "borderline hysteria." He backed up his charge by referring to a study by the Centers for Disease Control. There was only one problem. Well, actually there were two problems. First, there was no CDC study. Second, Koop had signed a $1 million contract with WRP Corporation which makes (Surprise!) latex gloves. In addition, his contract, which called for Koop to give four speeches a year after he had submitted them to the company for "editing," entitled Koop to a five-year option to purchase 500,000 shares of the company's stock at a *1994* price and gave him a percentage of the net sales of a new line of nutrition products that WRP was entering. He had somehow forgotten to mention these connections both when he spoke to Dr. Rosenstock and when he testified before the congressional committee.[14] The *Chicago Tribune* asked in an editorial whether the esteemed ex-Surgeon General was "a doctor or a shill." The *Trib* described the "blatant conflict of interest" as "shocking," but what was "More shocking still is his apparent inability to understand what the problem is."[15]

By the mid-1990s, it was hard to keep track of Koop's multifarious ventures without a scorecard, or at least a copy of the *Wall Street Journal.* The corporation names were different, but the story was always the same. ABC Inc., a gobbledygook provider that manufactures diet supplements on the side, proudly announced that Dr. C. Everett Koop, former Surgeon General of the United States, had joined its board of directors. This gave ABC Inc. instant cachet; news accounts noted Koop's sterling reputation for integrity, and the doctor allowed as how he was constantly being tempted with multimillion dollar offers to endorse product X and company Y, but he, no mere mortal, turned them all down, indignantly. For he would never ever trade upon the trust he had earned from the American people. However, after months of investigation, Dr. Koop had determined that ABC, Inc. was no run-of-the-mill money-grubbing capitalist concern: it was noble, it was pure, it was on the verge of finding a miracle cure for [FILL IN DISEASE]. So he had accepted ABC Inc.'s offer to sit on its board. He preferred not to disclose his compensation. Money was the furthest thing from his mind: we're talking about healthcare, about lives, for goodness sake—money never even entered the calculus of Koop's decision. And, oh, by the way, ABC Inc. was on the cutting edge of empowering consumers to blah, blah, blah.

All things considered, buying a piece of Koop was not a bad investment. He acted as a kind of Good Housekeeping seal of approval, at least the first dozen or so times he lent his name to a venture. For example, when First Circle Medical Inc. of Minneapolis undertook to raise funds for the development of experimental "hyperthermia" technology, it needed a quick infusion of credibility just as much as it needed the cash. Hyperthermia, an outgrowth of what is sometimes known as "fever therapy," raises the patient's core body temperature to almost 108 degrees Fahrenheit, whereupon doctors remove small amounts of the patient's blood, heat it, and return it to the body. The hope is that hyperthermia may be a way to combat AIDS, hepatitis C, and some cancers. That is the hope, at all events, for hyperthermia dates to the fourth century B.C. and has yet to fulfill its promise.

In January 1998, First Circle Medical Inc. announced that its board of directors had corralled a prize celebrity, C. Everett Koop. "He has an incredible mind to look at things with a solid foundation," First Circle Medical president Karl Groth told *Medical Industry Today*, "He brings a very strong credibility to hyperthermia."[16] He also carried along an ego so large that it almost literally squeezed out the rest of the board. In First Circle's "Board of Directors Profiles," chairman Alan J. Hamel, cofounder of the company, is profiled in seven lines; Dr. Bonnie Baskin, who founded ViroMed Laboratories, checks in at twelve lines; the modest Katherine A. Bjorkman is explained in but six lines (Scandinavian self-effacement, no doubt); Rudy A. Mazzocchi, CEO of Microvena Corp., is satisfied with ten lines. Swamping them like the tidal wave that overturned the *Poseidon* is Dr. C. Everett Koop, who consumes ninety-eight lines in a display of world-class insecurity.[17] (Did I ever tell you I got an A in Chem 101 at Dartmouth in 1935? . . .)

True to form, Koop declared that he had "examined the company's performance and the people involved"[18] before hopping aboard First Circle. He wanted to "find out if this is efficacious with big diseases," a spokesman said. The fact that First Circle Medical's work "dovetails" with that done by BioPure was also a consideration, conceded Koop: BioPure's blood substitute could well be used in raising a patient's body temperature, in which case the bank account of Dr. Koop would hit the biotech daily double.

First Circle Medical president Groth said that Koop's advice to his company would be "on the scientific side,"[19] a remark that is every bit as accurate as a D.C. lobbying firm's announcement that former Senator Smith is being retained for his keen mind and legislative acumen. The Koops and senators-turned-lobbyists of our nation open doors and make deals; otherwise, what good are they? Visitors to First Circle

Medical research facilities are no likelier to find Dr. Koop in a lab coat, fiddling with a test tube and microscope, than they are to find Senator Smith burning the midnight oil while crafting precise legislative language. That job is for the technicians: the lawyers and doctors who do the real work. C. Everett Koop left their ranks the day he answered that phone call from Senator Helms's office.

In any event, First Circle Medical got what it wanted right off the bat. Press accounts called Koop "a big-name ally."[20] His decision "to lend his reputation and clout" to First Circle Medical means that its hyperthermic ambitions are "more than a pipedream." (An unfortunate image, given the doctor's anti-tobacco fanaticism and his history of pipe smoking.) Koop's "urgency" about developing hypertheria technology "is compelling from both a humanitarian and a market standpoint,"[21] gushed one press rhapsodist. This is the best of both worlds, publicity-wise, for the company: Koop lends humanitarian gloss while endowing it with commercial potential.

Flitting from corporate board to corporate board, Chick also alighted on Bionutrics, not to be confused with BioPure. The company was incorporated in Nevada in 1990 with a stated goal "to pursue a marriage between food and drugs." But isn't this what Jerry Garcia and Cass Elliott sought? you ask. Not exactly. The Phoenix-based Bionutrics develops and markets dietary supplements—theoretically it does, for in practice the company keeps rolling Edsels off its line. A rice bran facility opened in Louisiana—and was sold for much-needed cash. A ballyhooed cardiovascular dietary supplement, EvolvE, flopped. Half of the company's 100 employees were canned. By 1999, Bionutrics was casting about for "functional nutrition products" that might reverse its monthly negative cash flow of $1 million. It was pinning its hopes on "favorable consumer shifts"[22] toward dietary supplements. These shifts are the result, in part, of the drumbeat of the nutrition nannies. Dr. Koop's projects, from Shape Up America! to Bionutrics, were a model of integration. And given that the FDA monitors the claims of those who market dietary supplements, Bionutrics made a shrewd investment in bringing aboard that old friend of the regulators, C. Everett Koop.

EvolvE, introduced in 1997 as Bionutrics' first product, was marketed as a cholesterol-fighter. The targeted audience was "consumers concerned about nutrition and health,"[23] making it a good Koop fit, but wait . . . hadn't the doctor disparaged the importance of his own cholesterol readings, implying that the cholesterol scare was so much wind? What was he doing on the board—what was he doing as a major shareholder—of a company whose first product, whose primary product, was an anti-cholesterol drug? Well, he might just want to claim ignorance. The company's February 25, 1999 notice to shareholders noted that Dr. Koop and one other board member were truant for more than one-quarter of the company's fiscal year 1998 meetings.[24]

Dr. Koop joined the Bionutrics board of directors on Halloween 1995, coming in with Milton Okin, founder of Weight Watchers and owner of a mail-order vitamin business. The more America tried to shape up, the richer these fellows got. Upon joining the board, Koop received an option to purchase 180,000 shares of Bionutrics stock at $1.50 a share. By February 1998, he owned 203,333 shares, or 1.1 percent of the company. But then the going got tough, and Koop got selling. One year later, on March 1, 1999, the doctor owned just 26,667 shares. The company concedes that a "thin market" for its stock has led to "extreme price and volume fluctuations."[25] Traded on the Nasdaq SmallCap Market, Bionutrics stock ranged between $14.625 per share in the second quarter of fiscal year 1997 to barely over $1 per share in early 1999. No wonder Koop quit going to meetings.

Koop also acts as an advisor to Neurocrine Biosciences, a San Diego-based neuroimmunology company that is pursuing research that may eventually benefit those who suffer from multiple sclerosis, type 1 diabetes, Alzheimer's Disease, and numerous other illnesses. Doing the Lord's work, you might say, and ingeniously so, at least if the many "Buy" recommendations from investment firms can be trusted.

The Koop connection is hard to understand, at first: what putative expertise does he bring to Neurocrine, other than his celebrity and his ability and willingness to throw his weight around with regulatory agencies? But in fact the hortatory head of Shape Up America! fits rather nicely in one Neurocrine niche: the search for an anti-obesity drug.

Corticotropin releasing factor (CRF), a brain hormone discovered in 1981, regulates the body's response to stress. Clinical tests have revealed that CRF antagonists can decrease appetite in "a genetically mutant strain of obese animals,"[26] which may sound like a polite description of NFL offensive linemen but is not. Assuming unpleasant side effects can ever be controlled—a big assumption—CRF antagonists may be the fen-phen of the new millennium. Or should we say a fen-phen that fulfills its promise.

So you see, Dr. Koop may be thought to be "drumming up business" for Neurocrine's Next Big Drug. "Commercial success for anti-obesity agents would be in the hundreds of millions"[27] of dollars, according to Gruntal & Co., a Wall Street investment research firm. (Eli Lilly is Neurocrine's partner in obesity drug development, one of three such "strategic alliances" the company has entered with pharmaceutical giants, the other partners being Janssen, a subsidiary of Johnson & Johnson, and Novartis.)

It may seem that C. Everett Koop has the golden touch, though what turns to gold is usually his bank account, not necessarily the products he hawks. For his most public venture was a colossal and humiliating flop—albeit one that made Koop ever richer.

In 1994, Time Life announced, with fanfare usually reserved for treaties of peace or landings on the moon, that something called Time Life Medical would produce a series of medical videotapes with Dr. C. Everett Koop, the revered former surgeon general. These tapes—seventy-five were envisioned—would cost $19.95 and be sold primarily in pharmacies. "This initiative merges the medical leadership of Dr. Koop with the marketing savvy of Time Life Inc., a brand name synonymous with high quality, accessible information throughout the world,"[28] averred John M. Fahey, president and CEO of Time Life Inc. If only he knew.

Lured by the magical Koop name, the heaviest hitters on Wall Street lined up behind the tapes: not only Time but E.W. Scripps, an affiliate of Lazard Freres & Co., and "numerous smaller investors" kicked in $40 million for this can't-miss project. The tapes were the brainchild of one J. Keith Green, who repeated, mantra-like, "One baby boomer turns 50 every 7.6 seconds," as if the fairly well-known fact that people age somehow guaranteed a rush on videotapes at Rite-Aid. Green foresaw $50 million in sales within four years. Green was loathed by those who had worked on previous projects with him: around the cutthroat world of advertising he was known as "the Darth Vader of Advertising."

Reeling from a chain of setbacks, Green hit upon medical videos as a fertile field for money growing. But he needed a hook; he needed a gimmick to interest the big boys. Finally, he wangled an introduction to Dr. Koop, and he got right to the point: "Time Life has a reputation for accuracy. You have a reputation for honesty and integrity. That's a brand."

That's a brand. The vaunted probity, rectitude, and fearlessness that Dr. Koop had cultivated were . . . a brand. So was the good doctor insulted by this vulgarian from the advertising world who dared compare his reputation to a dog food label? If he was, Green's offer of $750,000 a year to serve as board chairman of Time Life Medical made everything all right.

Each half-hour tapes would feature the somber Dr. Koop explaining various medical problems: coronary heart disease, prostate cancer, diabetes, depression, breast cancer. Anchoring the broadcasts was Linda Ellerbee, the smug network newsreader. Pharmacies were targeted as the primary site of sales. After all, who goes to the pharmacy? Sick people. What do they do at the pharmacy? Wait around for their prescriptions to be filled. So why not place a rack of informative videos about their medical conditions right in front of the milling millions in the nation's pharmacies? Who could resist plunking down twenty bucks for an impulse purchase of a video about what ails you?

Within a year, cameras were rolling. Rather than produce three or four videos at first, working out the kinks both creatively and commercially, Green and Koop plunged ahead, completing thirty Koop videos by October 1995. The sets were opulent; Green demanded a "Jeffersonian" backdrop, by which he did not mean a set dedicated to the principles of agrarian liberty. No, he wanted majesty; he wanted the appearance of "the information hub of the greatest patient-education center there was." For $375,000, Koop had a two-tiered information hub along which to stroll and act authoritative.

Doubters were ignored: these small-minded nabobs of negativism were the sort who said man would never walk on the moon! So with a lavish advertising campaign, Time Life Medical launched its thirty Dr. Koop videos in early 1996. All the stops were pulled out: *Time* published the aforementioned special health edition, featuring the star of its videos; something called the Vesalius Trust for Visual Communications in the Health Sciences awarded Koop and Time Life Medical "the prestigious Frank Netter Award for Outstanding Contribution to Medical Education."

J. Keith Green sat back and waited for the millions to wash over him. And waited. For as the *Wall Street Journal* reported, "Sales figures were disastrous." No one wanted to buy the damned things! They sat there in the middle of the store, taking up racks that might better be used to hawk comic books, bunion medications, anything. Pharmacies demanded their money back. Green had trouble meeting his payroll. And when that happened, Chick flew the coop. He resigned from the board of Time Life Medical—which had been created to accommodate him in the first place. Time, unwilling to squander more millions and further sully its name, pulled out.

By the time the *Wall Street Journal* picked over the bones in 1997, the project was $25 million in debt, Linda Ellerbee was complaining that she had reduced her fee to anchor the unseen videos—Dr. Koop's annual fee of $750,000 was not a cut rate, as Linda must have learned to her dismay—and enough unsold tapes were piled up in warehouses to fill craters on the moon. "We regret that the original vision for the company was not realized,"[29] is all Time Inc. had to say about the matter, in a whale of an understatement.

So did C. Everett Koop take this failure like a man, or at least mouth the conventional banalities about this being "a learning experience"? Please. No, he blamed Time for abandoning ship just before he was to do a video on smoking. The tobacco lobby—triumphant again!

You might think that a celebrity who can sucker Time-Life and an array of Wall Street firms into ponying up $40 million for a series of videos in which the unappetizing duo of C. Everett Koop and Linda Ellerbee talk about prostate cancer would be ineligible for government assistance. You might think that a man pulling down a $750,000 annual salary for one project—never mind the compensation from the various boards (and the stock options) on which he is a director, and the $25,000-a-speech gigs—would be ashamed to go begging for—well, insisting on—a government handout. You might think that a man who takes such obvious pleasure in donning the costume of a general—albeit a surgeon general—would be reluctant to put on the dress and tiara of the corporate welfare queen. But when there's money to be gathered, there is very little the voracious Dr. Koop will not do.

We have already seen the cozy alliance effected by Dr. Koop and the Clintons: he shilled for the ill-fated health plan, while Hillary promoted Shape Up America! and Bill arranged for the good doctor's bones to be interred at Arlington National Cemetery. But Koop being Koop, the currency of this alliance was not simply favors and speeches. Money changed hands as well. The loot went from the hapless U.S. taxpayer—you remember her: that corpulent crapulent consumer of cheeseburgers and beer, the only known antidote to which is fen-phen or whatever diet drug Koop, Inc. is pushing this week—to the Koop Foundation, Incorporated (KFI).

Like all organizations these days, KFI had a mission: "Improve Health . . . Fight Disease . . . Through the broad application of Health Informatics."[30] Okay, so it's not "To boldly go where no man has gone before," but in the ego department, the captain of the *U.S.S. Enterprise* had nothing on the founder of the KFI.

By the admission of its own propagandists, the Koop Foundation was founded at the request of Vice President Albert Gore, Jr. As the KFI tells it, "In December of 1993, Vice President Al Gore asked C. Everett Koop, MD to help identify and stimulate the private sector leadership that would make the greatest impact on building the health component of the National Information Infrastructure (NII)."[31] Just why the private sector had to be "stimulated" is a matter on which partisans of different political faiths will differ, but why Koop? Why December 1993?

Might the timing have anything to do with the fact that three months earlier, in September 1993, Dr. Koop had delivered his aforementioned gush that President Clinton had "done more for health care reform in the past four months than all of his living predecessors put together"?[32] As Koop campaigned for Clinton care in 1994, his operatives were busy setting up the Koop Foundation. Its launching was accompanied by the usual techno-gobbledygook that so bewitches Vice President Gore, the man who once boasted that he had invented the Internet. "We can use high-tech to cut cost by investing dollars wisely in the right kind of medical information technology and in superhighways," said Koop. "This will provide better, more accessible healthcare at a lower cost for all of us."[33]

His prattle may as well have been written by a neoliberal software program. "Investing dollars wisely" is Clinton-Gore-speak for spending taxpayers' money. "Superhighways" are, well, *super*. Who can be against that? And "lower cost for all of us": hey, count us in.

What Koop did not say is that this "lower cost for all of us" was to be achieved through a $15 million grant to the Koop Foundation. (This is where "investing dollars wisely" comes in, no doubt.) Cutting through the bureaucratese, the Koop mission was to figure ways to streamline the flow of information among the various parties to healthcare, from provider to patient. It envisioned "huge databases," "automated clinical guidelines," "automated coding and patient tracking"[34]—the computerization of the medical industry. Whether this is good or bad—Koop had once been quoted as saying that the house-call ought to be revived, and it is hard to see a place for house-calls in the hyper-automated world of health informatics—this computerization had been proceeding apace for some years, quite without the "stimulation" of C. Everett Koop.

But $15 million buys a lot of macadamia nuts, so the KFI was born.

The grant was administered under the National Institutes of Standards and Technology (NIST)'s Advanced Technology Programs (ATP). Actually, the *grants* were. For the KFI was responsible for two projects: first was the Health Informatics Initiative (HII), the would-be streamliner of the healthcare data-flow. One stated purpose of the HII was to feed "the expanding commercial need for health information."[35] In other words, to subsidize health-care businesses. And as we shall see, long after this $15 million was spent, Dr. Koop had reaped far more money for himself than Uncle Sam's initial investment. But the KFI cannot be faulted for dishonesty: up front, it admitted that one of its "target outcomes" was "to exploit the emerging national information infrastructure (internet, www, etc.)."[36] And that it did.

A second KFI project, begun several months later with a $9.882 million NIST grant, was HOLON, or Health Object Library ON-line. This sought to "establish middleware architecture to facilitate creation and use of health informatics and telehealth applications,"[37] which is to say that it followed up on the HII. Thus the federal government subsidized the Koop Foundation in its effort to speed the dissemination of health-care information via new technologies—the same thing several dozen other companies had long been trying to do without picking the taxpayers' pockets in the process.

The applications of the HOLON project were positively prosaic: one central "focus" was getting "self-reported patient health and lifestyle data incorporated into clinical records."[38] Not a bad idea—but was almost $10 million of taxpayers' money essential to that less than herculean task?

Government's involvement with high-tech is an old story, going back through Apollo to the Manhattan Project, but the ATP was different, or so it claimed: its goal was "economic growth and . . . good jobs and quality of life." This was the Clinton administration, after all: these were *New Democrats*, for God's sake: this was Clinton and

Gore, not LBJ and HHH. Clinton-Gore Democrats didn't feed at the pork barrel—they *invested wisely*. "ATP=Industry-Driven,"[39] blared the NIST home page; "Research priorities for the ATP are set by industry, not government."[40] But wasn't it Vice President Gore who came to Dr. Koop and asked him to develop a health informatics system? Er, well, it's a "partnership"; indeed, the "ATP is a new model of government-industry cooperation."

The ATP became one of Vice President Gore's favorite schemes, a "unique partnership between government and private industry" to foster risky "projects with a high payoff for the nation as a whole."[41] If one defines "nation" as "C. Everett Koop," then you've got it.

Koop is nothing if not a quick study. He learned to talk the New Democrat lingo. The KFI, in a presentation to its federal sponsors about health informatics, noted that healthcare was the "[m]ost expensive industry and everything done on paper. 'Collect many times, use once'—a poor paradigm for 1995 healthcare."[42] Now, when you consider that the paperwork received from our FOIA request earned a couple of UPS handlers overtime pay, the federal government is perhaps not the most receptive audience for complaints about excessive paperwork. But "paradigm" is the kind of word that makes the bureaucratic head nod, and the KFI was breaking old paradigms and building new ones all over the place. It worked for "patient empowerment"; scaling the heights of technobabble, it saw "Infrastructure as an Enabling Technology Solution." Truly an idea for which men will lay down their lives!

The ATP awards "are made strictly on the basis of rigorous peer-reviewed competitions designed to select the proposals that are best qualified in terms of"[43] blah, blah, blah. But when the Vice President of the United States has asked a celebrity to apply for a federal grant, and that celebrity has lent his name—his *brand* name—to the First Family's most cherished cause, you can damn well bet that the grant will be awarded. And so it was.

As the Koop project geared up, a July 26, 1996 hearing on health informatics before the House Subcommittee on Human Resources and Intergovernmental Relations revealed that various private concerns were doing—with their own money—what the Koop-APT "partnership" was doing with your money. The HMO U.S. Health Care had recently "launched a $25 million consumer health information activity."[44] Patricia Taylor, director of Health Education and Human Service Information Systems of the General Accounting Office (their titles are never simple, are they?), told the subcommittee of numerous informatics projects, both private and public. Most were "very young, under 2 years old, and in very early stages of development."[45] Their aims spanned the firmament; their labors had met with varying degrees of success. Typical was Access Health, Inc., which "contracts with insurers, managed care programs, and employers to provide advice on illness prevention, disease management, and general health information to their enrollees and employees. The company employs close to 500 people, including nurses and technical support personnel; it reports that it has spent about $20 million on systems development over the last seven years."[46] Or about $5 million more than C. Everett Koop's foundation received from the American taxpayer to "facilitate" projects similar to what Access was already doing.

"Projects are monitored and can be terminated for cause before completion,"[47] warned the National Institutes of Standards and Technology. The KFI projects were not terminated but they were monitored, and they left enough of a paper trail to suggest that Koop was not exactly a model grantee. The authors of this book filed a Freedom of Information Act (FOIA) request for all available material on the two Koop grants; eight months later, some 5,424 pages of documents chockablock with incomprehensible bureaucratese arrived. They tell a disturbing story.

The NIST published its invitation for proposals for the Advanced Technology Program in the Federal Register of March 21, 1994, four months after Vice President Gore asked Dr. Koop to lead us into the twenty-first century. Some fifty-nine applications were received; 16 were awarded grants. For you baseball fans, that's a batting average of .271. Not bad, especially given the $70 million available for these ATPs. If you've no qualms about taking government money to do things that private concerns are already doing, you might want to put in your own application.

The C. Everett Koop Institute at Dartmouth College was awarded $14,741,491 in ATP funds for its project, which was to run from January 1, 1995 to December 31, 1997. It was to be a joint venture: the Koop Institute's original partners included AT&T (surely a company in dire need of federal subsidy) and eleven other entities, mostly software companies, among them Oracle Corp., Logicon, Inc., and Meta Software. The total cost of this matching-grant project would be

$29,505,672. (The final cost turned out to be $30,868,943.) The grants specialist first assigned to the case was Donna Jean Garrett, who might have preferred to spend the lifetime of this grant banging her head against the wall, walking over a continent of hot coals, or engaged in some other activity more pleasurable than dealing with the Koop Institute.

The early paperwork raised one red flag: Booz, Allen & Hamilton, a technology consulting firm, had recently been punished for ripping off the government. As the firm admitted in paperwork filed for the Koop project:

> On August 20, 1993, after cooperating with the U.S. Attorney's Office for the Middle District of North Carolina, Booz, Allen pled guilty to two counts of filing false claims in violation of 18 U.S.C. Sec. 287 in connection with time charging irregularities, which occurred in the conduct of assignments under subcontract to the U.S. Environmental Protection Agency in 1988 and 1989.
>
> Booz, Allen paid a fine and restitution to the Government. The Firm entered into a compliance agreement with EPA, which provides that Booz, Allen will not be suspended or debarred.

Reassuringly, Booz, Allen noted that "[w]e have recently revised our time charging policy."[48] Well, okay, as long as you cross your heart and hope to die, stick a needle in your eye that you won't ever do *that* again.

As if this weren't enough, Dun & Bradstreet calculated Booz, Allen & Hamilton to have a risk factor of 9 on its scale of 1–9, with 9 representing the highest risk for investment. So one of the principal partners in the Koop grant was a high-risk company with a record of overcharging (not by enough, it would seem!): nonetheless, the grant was approved.

The paper trail is replete with complaints from the various bureaucratic monitors about Koop's intransigence. "Koop, those bad boys,"[49] as an early NIST e-mail refers to them. The first NIST grant officer, Donna Jean Garrett, is complaining in March 1995—right from the start—that she and her co-workers are at the end of their "rope with this Dave Taylor guy [Koop's lawyer]. They do not listen well. . . . Every time I turn around they have another change to a jv [joint venture] condition or term; and now they want to change the General Terms and Conditions!!! I told Mike [her boss] that I have 'nurtured' this group so much that they are on Vitamin C overload and their hair has now all fallen out!!!"[50] At one point she writes, "I have a call [into Koop] for narrative, justification, etc., but who knows if they get mad and yell at me!!!"[51]

Grants specialist Teresa Farris of NIST admonishes Dr. Michael D. McDonald of the Koop Foundation to stop advancing monies to its joint venture partners. "We realize in retrospect that we did not communicate our views of the use of the advancement of funds adequately,"[52] she tactfully writes, inviting a meeting.

Farris's superiors bent over backwards to coddle the Koop people; they excluded Farris from meetings, prompting her to protest, "Gwen [Simpson, a colleague] and I are trying to get Koop used to a new management style over here and indirectly you have sent a message to Koop that we do not function as a team."[53] Gwen Simpson writes to Farris that their exclusion is intended to keep potentially irksome overseers "out of the picture as far as KOOP is concerned. It's no wonder KOOP feels they can dictate to us. I can see we are going to have a difficult time with the KOOP awards."[54]

You can say that again, Gwen.

Time and again higher-ups at NIST let the little things—or not so little things—pass. The grant specialists were sometimes disarmingly candid in their remarks about the incompetence of their bosses, and it is not our purpose to get good people into hot water by publicizing these criticisms. Nonetheless, Koop got the kid glove treatment, the sort you'd expect to be given to . . . well, to a friend of the First Lady and the Vice President.

The necessary papers were always being filed late, if at all. Reports were missing. Advances were requested—or demanded. They asked for, and got, an extra six months to complete the project. "That project has a lot of problems to be resolved,"[55] grouses one NIST inspector.

Koop was always taking on new joint venture partners and losing others and not bothering to tell the increasingly exasperated grant-monitors what was going on. AT&T dropped out. SRA (Systems Research and Applications Corporation) dropped out. Logicon dropped out. Western Consortium for Public Health dropped out. Science Applications International Corporation dropped out. Beth Israel Hospital was a jv for months without NIST's approval. "[T]hey can not keep shuffling jv members back and forth,"[56] complains Donna Jean Garrett, to no effect. For they are Koop, and they will do as they please, and if you don't like it, well . . . hey, take that cigarette out of your mouth! Lose the potato chips! Any more sass and it's off to the Dietary Re-education Camp for you, you meddlesome bureaucrat. . . . On occasion, Koop was mildly disciplined. "I have denied the request for retroactive approval," wrote grants specialist Teresa Farris. "The Grants Office does not just 'rubber stamp' retroactive approvals."[57]

The would-be watchdogs at NIST were gently advised to loosen their grip. "Donna Jean," wrote one, "please don't get the impression that you should not raise issues such as this [irregularities in the Koop project]. It is essential that you speak up whenever you see something that doesn't look right to you and make us think twice about what we are doing."[58]

So they thought twice and let Koop slide through. "I will back down and support [*sic*] program if you all feel it is insignificant,"[59] replies Garrett.

A disastrous dispute over accounting and financial management between NIST and Oracle, the database software provider, very nearly destroyed the project before it even began. NIST stopped payment to Oracle, a key member of the team, until these issues were resolved. "The Oracle Issue Impacted this project to a point that major tasks were left undone from one year to the next,"[60] wrote Teresa Farris in an April 1997 e-mail that was blacked out by censorious editors of our FOIA request—but when the sun shines just right on the upheld paper, the words are legible. (Memo to Censor: buy a new magic marker.)

The second Koop grant, for the HOLON project, was no different. From September 1995, when the grant was announced, joint venture partners dropped out left and right. The amount involved was somewhat less—the feds kicked in $9.882 million toward a $19.973 million project—but the problems were just as pervasive.

Rice University dropped out of HOLON. Southern New England Telephone Company followed suit. "[W]ithdrawals have created a timeline performance issue for some areas of the project,"[61] explained the Koop Foundation in a language that looks suspiciously like English. This was by way of requesting an extension for the completion of HOLON. Again, the files are littered with notes from grant specialists about the special treatment Koop seems to be receiving. "[I]t concerned me that IntelliTek [a jv] could withdraw so late in the project and request an effective date back to the project origination date," wrote Teresa Farris in a note dated August 1, 1998. But "BJ [her superior] seemed to be fine with this occurrence."[62]

Oracle was also a member of HOLON. Once the lawyers negotiated

Oracle back onto the gravy train, it joined such other worthy almoners as Time Warner Cable at the feast: both pledged to integrate HOLON concepts into their products. Other companies have to pay research and development costs for such advances; the fortunate few can stick Uncle Sam with the R&D bill.

Two years into the grants, in 1997, the Koop people imperiously announced that they were transferring the two ATP projects from the Koop Foundation, the New Hampshire-based not-for-profit which was the awardee of the grants, to a new Maryland-based not-for-profit called The Health Initiatives Foundation, Inc. (HIFI).

An unusual request, but it was granted. For what choice did NIST have?

The KFI was based in Rockville, Maryland, a Beltway suburb, which was the source of some confusion to those who were administering the grant. After all, the original health informatics grantee was the Koop Foundation at Dartmouth College, which when last we checked was located in New Hampshire.

"[I]s the Koop location at Dartmouth College doing R&D and getting ATP funding on the Koop I project?" one puzzled grant specialist asked a superior. "Is this a central location for the Koop Foundation? I know they submitted the proposal, but that local Koop group [in a Beltway office in Maryland] is administering [*sic*] project. . . . Anything you can suggest re 'public' description of what the NH folks are doing on project . . . would be very helpful."[63]

Anything turned out to be nothing. "The bottom line is that both Koop ATP [*sic*] are run out of the Shady Grove [Maryland] Office, and nothing really is happening in NH,"[64] replied the superior. New Hampshire looked good on the application—the feds like to distribute pork to the hinterlands now and then—but Koop is a Beltway production, and this was Beltway work. Besides, New Hampshire, Maryland: what's the difference to a National Celebrity, the Conscience of His Country, a . . . TV Man?

Problems at the Koop Foundation ran deep. In October 1998, an e-mail went out from KFI head honcho Detlev "Doug" Foellmer to all the little satellites in the Koopian solar system. "The following communication has been received by the Koop Foundation Incorporated from Dr. Koop via counsel," Foellmer announced, as though he had just received a new papal bull. "KFI has been directed to disseminate this communication to interested and affected parties." The substance of the Koopian bull was that Dr. Michael D. McDonald of the Maryland office, whose title had been KFI director of HII, was now a nonperson.

The "counsel" referred to therein was Bruce A. Gunther, and his letter read, in part:

> As Dr. Koop's personal attorney, I have been directed by him to respond to certain information and, perhaps, misinformation which appear to be circulating regarding Dr. Koop's involvement in various organizations and initiatives. . . . Dr. Koop's foundation, The Koop Foundation Incorporated, has no present intention of either making or participating in any further ATP project submissions to NIST. . . . Dr. Koop has no business relationship with HIFI . . . and has no plans to become involved . . . in the future. . . . While Dr. Koop is generally supportive of Dr. Michael McDonald, Dr. Koop is not specifically endorsing any effort by Dr. McDonald or Dr. McDonald's related enterprises, nor is Dr. Koop a business associate of Dr. McDonald in any ventures.[65]

Well. HIFI was created by the Koop Foundation, but by this time the doctor had bigger fish to fry than the measly fare served up by NIST, and by humiliating his erstwhile associate McDonald in this manner he made it clear that his days of grant-getting were past. From here on in, the millions raked in by the Koop name were not to be shared with joint venture partners; no, it was time to graduate to the big board: the stock market, which would be so bullish on Koop that *he* would be in position to start funding health informatics out of his own pocket, if so preposterous a notion might even be considered.

The HOLON project was closed out in March 1999. The world would be the same. The health informatics project was closed out six months earlier, in September 1998, and while the experience was useful to Koop in immersing him in the technoworld, his joint venture partners seemed to consider it a failure. "One real problem," stated the NIST close-out summary, "was the lack of discussion by the members, on their own nickel, regarding the development of products and the commercialization of products."[66] Not only was Uncle Sam expected to fund the R&D, the corporate welfare queens even wanted him to set up marketing plans. Oh well: that, perhaps, is a project for the Gore administration.

By the time the *New York Times* headlined Koop jesting, "I've gone commercial,"[67] it may as well have announced that the Pope was Catholic. Nevertheless, the newspaper of record treated this Koop admission as just another act in a life of selfless service. This was no sell-out: he was doing it *for the children*. The *Times* visited the Koop

Institute, based at the doctor's alma mater of Dartmouth. The Institute, which once appeared to be the major planet, if not the sun, of the Koop solar system, has been relegated to a far smaller role—say, as one of the smaller moons of Uranus. It was founded in 1992 to "create a new kind of medical student, dedicated to promoting community health and preventing disease, sensitive to the social and economic circumstances of patients, and motivated by humanitarian values rather than greed."[68] (Yes, in 1992 Dr. Koop was denouncing "greed." But men change their minds.) Under the Koop influence, aspiring physicians at the Dartmouth Medical School were no longer to be money-grubbing specialists who ignore the "human side" of health care. They would connect with real people by giving programs in the schools and advising indigent families (not, presumably, to go out and blow their last dollars on Time Life's C. Everett Koop videos).

The Institute sponsors lectures, a perpetual rain of anti-tobacco propaganda, and a few unconventional approaches to better health care. The last time we logged on to the website (http://www.koop.dartmouth.edu/), two of the five "Latest from the Institute" offerings were "Poetry readings by Partridge Boswell" and "Poetry Readings by Verandah Porche." No, we are not making those names up. Two of the remaining three "latest" Koop Institute features were "Confronting Tobacco" and "Dr. Koop: Perspective on the Tobacco Wars." There was also artwork (portraits of psychiatric ward patients) and "The Adventures of Fall-Down Brown," in which an eight-year-old boy learns about bicycle and roller-blading safety, germs, and "the wonderful similarities and differences that help to make humanity what it is today."[69]

The stern visage of Dr. Koop is never far and always warning us about the epidemic of the week. "We stand at the precipice of a grave threat to our public health," begins one typical "Important Message from Dr. Koop." It might make an amusing parlor game to guess *which* grave threat he is talking about. No, it's not AIDS, for "unless we do something about it soon, it will kill more people than AIDS."[70] Besides, AIDS was yesterday's epidemic; AIDS was so eighties, and we've all moved on. To end the suspense, this time the grave threat was Hepatitis C. A killer, to be sure, and not joke material, but do we really need *this*?: "The Koop Institute's graphic artists and designers produced animations and games about Hepatitis C, as well as two illustrated storybooks for children."[71]

The whole thing is slightly surreal, though no more so than The Koop Village, one of those virtual communities—which is to say artificial, unreal, and insubstantial communities—so beloved of those rootless national political creatures (Koop, the Clintons, Gore) who, having forsaken real community, seek its simulacrum in high-tech gimmickry. Located on the World Wide Web, the Koop Village has the appearance of a nineteenth-century New England village of the sort found around Dartmouth. Click onto a building and you're in a meeting room, where you can chat about Hepatitis C or the iniquity of the tobacco industry or any of a thousand topics of the sort that no actual New England villager of the nineteenth century would dream of broaching.

To be fair, the Institute does do some good work. Its "Take Time to Talk" brochure encourages greater communication between doctor and patient. A worthy goal, surely, though it is instructive to note that "Take Time to Talk" is funded by Pharmacia and Upjohn—pharmaceutical giants scrubbing Koop's back as he has scrubbed theirs.

The reporter doing the *New York Times* puff piece about Koop "going commercial" was careful to set the Dartmouth College students in the story "[c]rammed into a small back room"—the implication being that this is a shoestring operation staffed by dedicated idealistic kids who are doing it all *for the children*. The busybody students were producing a propaganda film pitting the evil Smoking Joe Moose, who is "trying to take over the world with the most addictive cigarette ever known," against "a character who bears a striking resemblance to the former surgeon general" and is trying to take over the world . . . no, cut that last part. He may well be trying to take over the world, or at least break us to his will, but that is most emphatically *not* in the script.

The fawning *Times* reporter went on to describe Dr. Koop's web page (http://www.drkoop.com), which had just been launched in December 1998, and which "offers free medical and health information about diseases, treatment, and medication options"—in other words, information you can find in any of a hundred books or web pages. Within two months of the creation of the web page, 15 hospitals had ponied up $100,000 each for room on drkoop.com. More followed soon thereafter. Pharmaceutical companies got in on the act, for among drkoop.com's services was the linkage of customers with pharmacies and online drugstores. The manufacturers of Nicorette gum sponsor

"Tackling Tobacco," which they hope you will do with their product. But however much he might joke about going commercial—a flash or two of self-deprecating wit is always good p.r.—Koop is never far from striking the Pose of Piety. He told the reporter that he was offered $1 million to endorse a cereal. "That I would not do,"[72] he thundered, as $1.5 million in hospital advertising blinked from his web site. But within months, drkoop.com would make its eponym rich beyond his wildest imaginings.

Unlike many octogenarians, Koop has embraced the computer with all the ardor of young love. And why not? The industry has been very, very good to him. Before the Koop Village darkened the nation's monitors, IBM "partnered," as they say in press release-speak, with the ill-fated Time Life Medical to create a Time Life Medical Center "virtual building" within the IBM Health Village. This was where virtual consumers were to gather virtual information about their actual diseases, but, alas, Time Life Medical is no more, having attracted virtually no customers for its prime product, the video line.

Koop also served on the board of directors of A.D.A.M. (Animated Dissection of Anatomy for Medicine) Software, Inc., from 1994 until 1997, when "pressing commitments"[73]—that is, the chance to make lots more elsewhere—necessitated his resignation. A.D.A.M. was classically Koopian: in April 1996, just three months before Koop felt the press of other commitments, a holder of 1,000 shares of A.D.A.M. common stock filed a class-action lawsuit against the company, alleging "violations of the Georgia Securities Act and negligent misrepresentation arising out of alleged disclosure deficiencies in connection with the Company's initial public offering."[74] To which A.D.A.M. responded by taking a lead role in demanding federal legislation to nullify such state-court lawsuits. In asserting the power of the national government over the states, this was contrary to the spirit of federalism to which the Republicans were then paying lip service, but it was very much in the centralizing tradition of Dr. Koop. His influence, it seems, had survived even his resignation from the board.

Before the break with A.D.A.M., the software company had demonstrated its wares at a Koop-hosted forum at Dartmouth College. The audience included the Rube Goldberg of the Clinton administration, Ira Magaziner, director of the ill-starred Health Care Task Force. Bringing business and government together: it's a lucrative job, but somebody's got to do it.

IBM and A.D.A.M. were not the only stalwarts of the computer industry to court Koop. In October 1998, visions of the wired millions glowing in his eyes, Dr. C. Everett Koop joined Andy Grove, chairman of Intel Corp., the chip and computer-manufacturing giant, to celebrate Internet Health Day at the Hyatt Embarcadero Hotel in San Francisco. There was much high-flown talk of how computers were the next great tool in the doctor's bag: health, philosophized one techno-huckster, is "one area that touches the lives of virtually everyone,"[75] and who could possibly disagree with that?

Grove hummed the buzzwords like a queen bee. He imagined "a futuristic bustling bazaar of online medical analysis where patients can become educated and empowered."[76] Whether we call this new Internet niche e-health or health informatics, only time and the market will tell us how profitable an idea it is.

Intel used the occasion to publicize its investment in several on-line health information ventures; as the *Los Angeles Times* noted, "Intel hopes a tremendous number of new consumers will want to buy Intel-based Pcs."[77] This is perfectly natural and healthy; what is not so natural is the involvement of America's doctor, the man who would never trade on his reputation, as a shill for Intel.

Just what was in it for Koop? Why play the scowling adman for Intel? Well, for one thing, there was www.drkoop.com, America's doctor's own site, via which doctors and physician groups can build their own websites, which are linked with Koop's site, "a reference source for consumers and doctors."[78]

Drkoop.com was run by what originally was known as Empower Health Corp., an Austin, Texas-based company founded in January 1997. It can be hard to keep all these corporate names straight: the Koop Foundation, the Koop Institute, the C. Everett Koop National Health Awards. But Empower was at the center of what the old populists used to call an interlocking directorate: a series of connections linking various corporations whose one common trait is the presence of Dr. C. Everett Koop.

Empower was "an Internet solutions and services company dedicated to empowering consumers to better manage their personal healthcare."[79] Or at least that's the p.r. version. "Empowerment" has become such a cant word, signifying everything and meaning nothing, intended to soothe conservatives (helping people do things for themselves!) *and* liberals (new tools for the consumer!) alike, that one should look askance at anyone who uses it. Empower began life as, in large part, a software records company: the plan was to "develop technologies that will revolutionize the way people manage their health care, by providing them with a wealth of on-line information and opportunities for interaction."[80] (Sounds almost exactly like a certain National Institutes of Standards project?) Central to Empower was a "personalized medical record system." But when that failed to fire many imaginations, the company married itself to that last refuge of the get-rich-quickies—the Internet.

In 1998, Superior Consultant Holdings Corporation, an immodestly named provider of Web services, entered a "strategic relationship"[81] with Empower Health Corporation. Superior acquired a "minority equity stake"[82] in Empower; in return, it agreed to provide Empower with software services, systems integration, and manifold duties sheltered under the capacious umbrella of "consulting." Richard Helppie, chairman, president, and CEO of Superior (the Superior superior), joined the board of directors of Empower Health Corp. to "lend my support to Dr. Koop and the management team at Empower Health to carry out their mission of empowering consumers to actively manage their healthcare needs."[83] He has the lingo down, anyway: empower consumers, actively manage—it's as though Newt Gingrich came back as a CEO. And yes, he also uses the phrase "cutting edge."

You stroke me, I'll stroke you: simultaneously, Dr. Koop joined the board of directors of Superior: he, too, looked "forward to partnering with Superior to empower consumers to actively manage their healthcare needs."[84] (Perhaps Shape Up America!'s next crusade could be aimed at reducing excess jargon.)

Health Data Network News translated the Superior-Empower marriage into the vernacular. Superior was "[h]oping to capitalize on Koop's name recognition and shining reputation." (There's that reputation again. Can nothing dull its shine?) Despite Empower Health Corp.'s lack of a single client or product in May 1998, when Superior consummated the deal, Richard Helppie bought in because of the value of the Koop name: "When people go on the Internet, they're often not sure of the quality of the information they're getting. Dr. Koop is widely recognized and trusted by consumers. His personal credibility will make Empower Health's services a superior offering,"[85]—pun, we are sure, not intended.

Dr. Koop, by the way, purchased, as a perquisite of his position on the Board of Directors, 3,000 shares of Superior stock, which, as we write this (November 1999), was trading at about $12 per share. The granting of stock options "is an important method of rewarding and motivating management by aligning management's interests with those of the Company's stockholders,"[86] according to Superior's 1999 report to those same stockholders. Undeniably true—just as it is true that Koop is raking in riches every which way he turns: Superior buys into Empower and places him on its board, compensating him in stock whose value shoots up when the value of Empower (now named drkoop.com) goes through the roof. Nice work if you can get it.

Superior is a holdings corporation consisting of two subsidiaries: Superior Consultant Company, Inc., which services the healthcare industry, and Enterprise Consulting Group, Inc., which provides support to such other industries as education, entertainment (but do *they* know Morgan Fairchild?), and financial services. The vast majority of the Southfield, Michigan-based company's employees (almost three-quarters of 800–plus) are consultants. Whatever Superior's qualities, and we are sure there are many, felicity of language is not among them. For instance, the company cannot really mean it when its publicity material boasts, "our name represents our approach to clients, employees and business partners."[87] Ought it not, then, be called Supercilious Consultant Company? Or perhaps Haughty Holdings? And what deranged muse inspired CEO Richard Helppie to ask the question that sits on the tongues of millions: "If we can put a man on the moon, why can't we get a very good healthcare information system or construct a management structure that absolutely reduces costs and unquestionably improves quality?"[88]

Admit it: in the dead of night, when all is quiet but for the occasional chirp of a cricket, haven't you asked yourself the same question?

Visions of consumer empowerment dancing in its head, Superior and Empower powered up. So just what was this ugly duckling named Empower before it metamorphosed into the swan-like drkoop.com?

Being a Koop project, Empower was heavily subsidized by pharmaceutical giants. Its "Prevention Center," part of a general Health & Wellness area, offered information on fitness, safety (such as how to perform CPR, which is one of those skills better learned in person, on a dummy, than off a screen), nutrition, the ever-reliable stress management (which might have come in handy for the harried NIST monitors of Koop's grants), and, of course, "tackling tobacco addiction."[89] In all, it was a dubious melange of slogans and lectures and information readily available elsewhere. The Prevention Center also featured a Personal Drugstore, which was neither personal nor a drugstore but did allow users to research drug interactions. The privilege of sponsoring this (im)Personal (non)Drugstore fell to PCS Health Systems, Inc., the biggest pharmaceutical care management company in the country, managing 300 million prescriptions totaling $10 billion. (A company spokesman fastidiously pointed out that just because a firm advertises on the Koop Web site doesn't mean that Koop endorses the product. Which claim is at odds with the implied cachet that comes with having your brand name next to one of the most valuable brand names in America—no, not Miller or Trojan, but Dr. Koop.)

Old habits—especially the exercise of condemnatory power—die hard. Though he no longer wears the uniform, Dr. Koop has been reluctant to part with the tools of the tyrant. Among the first projects he undertook on his Web site was . . . a review of every *other* Web site devoted to health. "There are 12,000 health sites on the Internet," he said, "and patients have no way to know if they are getting right or wrong information."[90] About, presumably, such matters as the non-link between eating fat and breast cancer. Like a humorless Roger Ebert (minus about forty years of inhaling Junior Mints and tubs of hot buttered popcorn), Dr. Koop—or, more probably, the flunky who acts in his name—rates the approved Web sites on a scale of one to five stars. According to *U.S. News & World Report*, "Koop says if a site doesn't appear in his rating system, it isn't worth looking at."[91] Somehow it's comforting to know that age cannot dim, or even dent, a good case of megalomania.

The site also features *Good Morning, America* celebrity Dr. Nancy Snyderman, channels dedicated to men, women, children, and the aged, and over 1,700 health and "wellness" topics, wellness being healthspeak for empowerment. Information ranges from helpful (warning signs of diabetes) to, well, Nancy Snyderman's advice on how to use a thermometer—"the different types,"[92] as the site tactfully put it. Any wire story playing up the rotundity of Americans is a surefire hit on drkoop.com. A typical search turned up the following less than balanced headlines: "US Waistlines: Super Sized"; "Mom's beliefs may cause child obesity"; "New Weight Guidelines: 55% in US Too Fat"; "Diet drug helps keep weight off" (yeah, sure); "Even small weight loss helps heart"; "Obesity treatment: MDs often need training"; "Obesity may increase gum disease risk" . . . you get the idea. The gist of these stories, as Drs. James Hill and John Peters are quoted in "US Waistlines: Super Sized," is that "Health professionals, the general public, and policymakers have not recognized obesity as a serious threat to health. . . . [I]t remains low on the list of important public health problems."[93] Moving it up the list is a project not only of Dr. Koop but also of the Web site that bears his name.

The site's "Personal Drugstore" permits a user to refill prescriptions from pharmacies or online drugstores. It has "partnered," to use the lingo, with Health Resources Publishing Company, the nation's biggest publisher of pharmacy information newsletters; HRP publications will include information and Web directions to drkoop.com. "Access to information is the key to patient empowerment,"[94] explained Dr. Koop in March 1999, when the partnership was consummated. He pledges to provide "world-class information," another meaningless phrase that has become a verbal tic of big businesspersons. HRP labors on behalf of more than forty companies, mostly pharmaceutical giants, including Bristol Myers Squibb and Pharmacia & Upjohn—many of the same companies with which the ex-surgeon general has been in bed since he became an ex. Not for nothing is the Empower/drkoop.com CEO Donald W. Hackett, whose degree is in marketing.

The thing to remember about Empower, or so its officers assured the investing world, is that it was to be, above all, "consumer-centric."[95] If you are like most people, you will respond, "What does that mean?" But then if you are like most people, you avoided Empower as if it were a three-dollar bill.

Perhaps by "consumer-centric" the folks at Empower meant that Dr. Koop placed consumerism at the center of his personal universe. Certainly that's the impression one gets from even a casual browse of his Web site. "[L]et's say you want to take advantage of opportunities we offer to purchase things online,"[96] chirps Dr. Koop's Community's "About Us" page. Let's say, indeed.

Empower sold itself to potential advertisers with an aggressiveness seldom seen this side of steroid-crazed jockdom. Its Web site offered "an unparalleled opportunity to reach healthcare consumers" (a rather bloodless euphemism for sick people). "There is not better [*sic*] opportunity on the Internet to reach such a targeted Health conscious audience."[97]

Its centerpiece, Dr. Koop's Community, provided access to disease and treatment information. The "community"—another word that has been stripped of meaning—was factitious: this was a community in the sense that watchers of a TV sit-com constitute a community. Nothing binds them—nothing substantial anyway—but it sounds so nice and cuddly and cozy to call anonymous consumers a "community."

Being a member of Dr. Koop's faux community means always having to say you're sorry for smoking. The site acts as a warehouse for any and all stories demonizing tobacco: on a typical day, one finds "Mom's smoking tied to child behavior problems"; "Call for grade school anti-smoking programs" (surely this is far too late: let us catch the tykes in preschool, if not the delivery room); "Increased risk of dementia in some smokers" (driven crazy by the incessant hounding by the surgeon general?); "Smoking linked to hearing loss"; and "Smoking linked to genital wart duration."[98] (Is there *anything* smoking is *not* linked to?)

A related project, Dr. Koop's Community Partner Program, offered "partnerships"—purchased in cash, not friendship—to hospitals and health-care organizations. Such partners as Memorial Health Services of Southern California and Tallahassee Memorial Healthcare became Community Partners, which enabled them to "create a co-branded, world-class local Web site that is dynamically linked with drkoop.com features, content, and resources."[99] In other words, they became conduits for Koop's Web site, giving the good doctor's advertisers and pharmaceutical sponsors more bang for the buck. Besides frequent use of the non-word "co-brand," Empower sold the Community Partner program using the lingo of a Madison Avenue firm hawking cat food: Morris eats his Friskies, the Pepsi Generation gulps its syrupy elixir, "Mike" Jordan chugalugs his Gatorade, sweaty jocks Just Do It in Nike sneakers, and a paragraph or two about your high-blood pressure pills are "co-branded with the award-winning drkoop.com brand and the Partner's [note the capital P—very classy] brand, improving image and enhancing loyalty." Brand loyalty, as in eat Cheerios, not Wheaties. Or perhaps this is a bad example, as Dr. Koop, in the days before he added the .com suffix, boasted that he would never ever take a million to endorse a cereal. (We now know that it wasn't the idea of an endorsement that he objected to, it was just that piddling million. As with the woman in the Winston Churchill story, we have established what he is—we're merely haggling about price.)

A second Empower product, Dr. Koop's Personal Record System, is a gussied-up version of those old sheets on which a person kept track of which shots he'd received. Keeping these records by keyboard rather than pen is the innovation here, though the cynical might call it more mindless techno-worship.

In any event, Empower lacked that certain indefinable Something that separates the wheat from the chaff, corporate-moniker-wise. So consumers were polled, markets were tested, and the number-crunchers of Bruskin-Goldring reported that almost six in ten Americans still knew who Dr. Koop was, and nearly five in ten considered him "the country's top health authority."[100] Never doubt the power of hype. As Donald Hackett, president and CEO of Empower Health Corp. said, "In the online healthcare world, it is imperative to establish a 'trustmark' for your users. Our site embodies that trust, and now, so will the name of our company."[101] Putting aside the question of just what the "trustmark" means, in March 1999 Empower Health Corp. became drkoop.com. Very high-tech, very lower-case, very '90s—which means, of course, that in time the gimmicky name will go the way of the Nehru jacket, the leisure suit, and Time Life Medical.

The advantage of the name drkoop.com, as Web site director Barbara Hansen told Matt Labash of the *Weekly Standard*, is that "out of the hopper, we have brand. We don't have to invent it."[102] There's that b-word again. A lifetime of sweat and sacrifice, of double shifts and harrowing operations, of stentorian pronouncements and prohibitionist labors, of red-eye flights and shrewd positioning, and eighty-some years later you are . . . a brand.

Hansen conceded that Koop is not the most active Web site eponym: "He's here about once a quarter," she guessed, a generous estimate that Koop soon corrected to "I've been there once."[103] He glances at the Web site that bears his name "about once a month." Yet he strenuously contests the charge that his activity is limited to cashing a paycheck. "I don't have my name on things with which I'm not involved," he says, indignantly. No, he's not logging on once a day to answer users' questions about diarrhea: "the best thing you could say is that I set the standards—it's too big for any one person to have his hand on everything." He does pledge to devote more time to the small-case drkoop "if I can ever get the rest of my life straightened out."[104]

Given that drkoop.com contains 70,000 pages, Dr. Dot.Com cannot be accused of micro-managing. But then as Labash notes, "One might patronize a Roy Rogers or KFC, but one would hardly expect to see the singing cowboy or Kentucky colonel—God rest their souls—standing over the fryer vats." It's brand that counts, and, like Roy and the Colonel, Koop "will live on" in cyberspace after his death, according to Hansen.

Whatever the fortifying effects of multiple martinis and macadamia nuts in whipped cream, Dr. Koop will not live forever. His expiry was "brought up quite a bit"[105] by potential investors, said Hansen, but their fears, evidently, were allayed on June 8, 1999, the day that will live in investor infamy, when we discovered that all that talk of "brand" was no mere hype; it was worth $84.4 million. A singular day it was, and one that foolish investors will yet rue. Nonetheless, somewhere in Icon Heaven, Roy and the Colonel were whistling with envy.

What a difference a name makes. In 1998, Empower Health Corp. lost $9 million; revenues were an astoundingly small $48,000. But "[w]hatever happens, Koop should do well,"[106] as *National Journal* noted smartly. In Empower's near-catastrophic first year of operation, as it staggered under $9 million in losses, Dr. Integrity pocketed $100,000 in salary, $95,000 in lecture fees, and $83,000 for the heavy lifting required as chairman of Empower's Board of Directors. Most importantly, he got 11 percent of its stock (over one million shares at first) and two percent of its revenue.

The ship was not exactly righted in the first quarter of 1999: revenues were $404,215, and losses were $4.3 million. The company did not forecast a profit in the near future. Then came the name change, and it was as though a rusty Pinto with a dropped engine and bald tires had, overnight, metamorphosed into a Mercedes. Suddenly, everyone wanted aboard.

The March 1999 public offering of stock in drkoop.com may not have seemed the bargain of the century to savvy investors, but the white elephant hoped to raise as much as $50 million. Bear Stearns & Company was the underwriter; the shares were to be traded on the Nasdaq stock market.

As it turned out, $50 million was too modest a goal by far. Investors, in the grips of .com fever, gave drkoop.com "a smashing Wall Street debut,"[107] in the words of the *Washington Post*. In its initial public offering of June 8, 1999, the company sold 9.4 million shares at $9 each, raising $84.4 million for a venture that had theretofore been a first-class dud. Shares were trading for as high as $20.25 on that first day before closing at $16 7/16. It seems that the taxpayers' modest investment in the Koop Foundation way back in 1994 had paid indirect dividends: the KFI project sought to "increase the level of access to health information,"[108] which is precisely what drkoop.com professed to do. From small things, baby, big things one day come.

"Reflecting Trust in Ex-Surgeon General"[109] is how the *Wall Street Journal* headline writers explained the extraordinary debut of drkoop.com. Given Empower's pathetic track record, investors were placing their full faith and trust in Dr. Koop. As Alan Abelson reported in *Barron*'s, "the business model mostly consists of exploiting the dickens out of Dr. Koop's universally familiar visage."[110] Almost two decades of public sanctimony had finally paid off.

So who profited from the drkoop.com boom? Dr. Koop minus the .com, of course, whose 2.5 million shares were worth as much as $60 million before the inevitable deflation of the company's balloon set in and he wound up Day One with paper wealth of $41 million dwarfing his company salary of $135,000. David Kessler joked that "Dr. Koop can now fund the entire [anti-tobacco] program," and Kessler knows the ravenously acquisitive Koop well enough to know what an outrageous jest that really is. Donald W. Hackett owned 7.1 million shares, Adventist Health System Sunbelt Healthcare Corp. had 2.8 million shares, and Superior Corp. had 5.2 million shares. The Empower-Superior marriage had borne rich fruit. (Also profiting—temporarily and illegally—was Dr. Nancy Snyderman, evidently a graduate of the C. Everett Koop school of money-grubbing. Her husband snatched up 1,650 shares of drkoop.com on June 8 for $9 and sold it a month later at $41.27 a share, making a tidy sum of $53,245. Alas, this violated insider-trading laws, so Dr. Snyderman and the Mr. had to return the loot.)

The wild ride wasn't over yet. Within a month of its smashing stock-market debut, drkoop.com zoomed to almost $37 a share with the announcement that it would shell out $89 million over five years to America Online Inc., which would feature Koop's site on five AOL sites. The crash was bound to come—but when? Perhaps only with the good doctor's death, which we hope will not come for many nag-ful years yet, but the straws are already in the wind, and a gale is blowing, not a calming zephyr.

On April Fool's Day 2000, a headline in the *Washington Post* heralded "Auditors Question drkoop.com's Health," and a few weeks later the *Post* announced "5 Months Left for drkoop.com." News of drkoop.com's death was decidedly premature, but the prognosis is not good if a share price of less than one dollar at which the stock traded in January 2001 is any indication of its future prospects.[111]

But if Koop's wealth expanded exponentially, he was, for the first time since his debut on the public stage as Dr. Koop, the avenging angel of the right-to-life movement, put in the pillory. "Hailed as a Surgeon General, Koop Critized on Web Ethics," ran the front-page headline in the *New York Times*. The article exposed Koop's receipt of from 2 to 4 percent of revenues derived from products sold at this site: after the piece appeared, this provision was eliminated from Koop's contract. The *Times* also noted drkoop.com's practice of recommending "the most innovative and advanced health care institutions across the country" with nary a mention of the $40,000 fee paid by those hospitals to be so denominated. This, too, was soon discontinued. The investigator disclosed that Koop was to receive a payment for each human guinea pig that Quintiles Transnational Corporation induced to participate in drug trials via the web site. Koop's defense: he had not profited because not a single person had volunteered. Which ought to raise questions in the minds of potential advertisers as to just how effective a transmitter of information drkoop.com really is.

Koop's reply to the *Times*' expose was classic: "I didn't go into drkoop.com to make money," he protested. "I did it to change the way that medicine is practiced." Just as patriotism is the last refuge of a scoundrel, the tobacco companies are the last refuge for Koop. "It is true there are people in my situation who could not receive a million-dollar grant and stay objective," he said in reference to the *Times'* noting his subsidization by the pharmaceutical industry. "But I do. I was approached by people who asked me if I would represent the side of tobacco in the tobacco settlement and I refused."[113] Yeah . . . sure.

Sensing a p.r. disaster, the web site went into spin mode. A message from Dr. Koop to site users noted that "the media is exploring the credibility of healthcare information supplied via the Internet, as well as the lines drawn between advertising and editorial content."[114] He added, "We at drkoop.com endorse this examination." Of course. And the typical arrestee appreciates and endorses the court's interest in determining the extent of his honesty.

But the bad press wouldn't stop. After Dr. Snyderman's insider-trading scam was revealed, Superior CEO Richard Helppie was caught at his own insider-trading game and required to return the profits therefrom.

Matt Labash noted that in Amsterdam, Dutch hookers advertise their wares under signs reading “te koop.” The translation is “For Sale.”[114] Which would be as good an epitaph as any when America’s most famous Dutchman goes to his final reward, in a cemetery other than that reserved for a nation’s heroes.

6

Epilogue: Chick and Hillary

"There, but for the Grace of God, goes God."
—Anonymous

Putting aside the uniform, the voice-of-God (or Chuck Heston) pronouncements, the self-glorification, the chiseling, the acquisitiveness, the eye for the main chance, and the multiple other annoying characteristics of the good Doctor Koop, perhaps the single flaw that stands out most—that makes so many good Americans grind their teeth when they see his mean mien or hear his hectoring voice—is his hypocrisy. He is a pharisee, a Tartuffe: a self-righteous blowhard so awash in his own piety and sanctimony that he's come to think it's holy water.

Maybe this explains the fact that he found his soulmate in Mrs. Clinton: the apostle of the "politics of meaning" who found time to make $100,000 on a token investment in cattle futures; the bleeding heart who made her reputation as a crusader for goo-goo causes but made her money as a hired gun for corporations; the woman whose supercilious glare says "I'm purer than you" and all the while she is pocketing fat fees from Tyson Chicken.

"I do whatever Dr. Koop tells me to do." A jesting remark, of course, but it implies no subservience, for Dr. Koop and Mrs. Clinton are soulmates. They'd act harmoniously even without pressure from the other. And Koop, unlike Mr. Clinton, never betrayed Hillary. Nor she him: even in such p.r. disasters as the Arlington National Cemetery fiasco, Hillary stuck by her man. Maybe she really was Tammy Wynette: not to the ne'er-do-well George Jones played by her snake of a husband, but to the upright C. Everett Koop, who, unlike Bill, mastered the art of imitating rectitude while he fleeced the sheep. If only Chick had been twenty-five years younger. . . .

Where will this all lead? In Hillary's case, to a long post-White House (and post-Bill?) career as a national nag, a pesterer, a hectoring hypocrite. In Koop's case, it led to the fattest bank account this side of the *Fortune* 500. And for the rest of us, well, it leads to more government controls on personal behavior, more excuses for extortionate levels of taxation and profligate federal spending, and liberties that are disappearing faster than a model on fen-phen.

Of course, according to those in the grip (and often in the pay) of diet mania, many, if not most Americans, are either obese or just a few Grand Slam breakfasts away from being so. We roll out of bed after a night of stertorous breathing, stumble down to the kitchen for a bag of donuts (when we really should be tossing off a five-mile run), get to work by the most exercise-averse way possible, and spend the day bumping into our fellow fatties while inhaling candy bars and dreaming about calorie-filled cheesecake.

Estimates of obesity in America have reached absurd proportions. The Koopian estimate of 58 million is bandied about regularly, though 70 million is gaining favor and 90 million is heard on occasion. Given the media taste for round numbers, our money is on 100 million fat Americans soon into the new millennium. The Centers for Disease Control now claim that one in five Americans is not just overweight, but *obese*. Southerners are particularly obtuse in their obesity: between 1991 and 1999, the obesity rate zoomed upward by 67.2 percent in the Southeast. In Georgia the increase was an incredible 101.8 percent. The health and fitness industry's culprits? Hot weather (who wants to go outdoors in sweltering heat?), suburban sprawl (all those KFCs in the strip mall just beyond the housing tract), and, in a Koopian echo, barriers to walking. "We don't have sidewalks that lead anywhere," fretted a dietitian with the Georgia Division of Public Health. So what is to be done? "A national strategy needed to combat obesity," according to the CDC.[1] And we know just the man to lead it.

If Southerners irritate the slim-is-beautiful crowd, black women must really drive them crazy. *Half* of all African-American women are adjudged obese. It should be noted that these figures did not decrease—America did not get fit and trim—during the eight-year reign of Surgeon General Koop. This is not to blame him for the national paunch, though given his expansive view of the powers of the federal government he may well regard this as a personal failure. In fact, federal government "health goals" had envisioned that by the year 2000 less than 20 percent of adults and 15 percent of adolescents would be categorized as obese. Americans have been extraordinarily uncooperative with the health police: they continue to gobble their mega-muffins and lick the fried chicken off their stubby fingers. The next step, or at least the attempted next step, will be coercive: taxes on fatty foods, bans on junk food. A plate of fettucine alfredo will cost more than a case of cognac; a lively black market in barbecued potato chips will spring up in response to their prohibition. The tradition of American liberty will be further trashed and traduced. But this is a story we have told elsewhere, in *The Food and Drink Police*.[2]

This may seem like hyperbole. A food and drink police? Come on, get real. Sure, revenuers and G-men and Volstead Act enforcers once roamed the land, a drink police of sorts, but the days of Prohibition are long past. We have learned our lesson that the federal government cannot, either morally or efficiently, interfere with what the American people choose to drink or eat. (Smoke is another matter.)

Or *is* smoke another matter? According to the *Journal of the National Cancer Institute,* "[a]dvocates of improved diet and exercise for better cancer prevention" have learned key lessons from "anti-tobacco advocates."[3] (One lesson they seem to have learned from the contemporary Chicken Littles of the second-hand-smoke wars is to ignore research that does not ratify their prejudices. Not the best lesson to have learned.)

The Nutrition Warriors have no desire to travel the "excruciatingly arduous and long path that anti-tobacco advocates had to travel"—another name for this excruciatingly arduous and long path is democracy. They want action *now.* And not just wimpy warning labels; they're demanding "prevention and control measures by government, the media, physicians, and educators."

The language of the Nutrition Warriors is sometimes elliptical, but we get their point. Advertising "the benefits of good nutrition or exercise aren't enough to change public behavior," laments the *Journal of the National Cancer Institute*. Adds Dr. Ernest L. Wynder, an early anti-tobacco crusader and now president of the American Health Foundation, "Asking patients to give up a habit they enjoy today for possible benefit in the future is a tough sell. Especially without social support." That phrase "social support" is ominous. For Wynder is emphatically *not* talking about a "keep up the good work" from your next-door neighbor. Instead, he urges physicians to become "political activists,"[4] with all that that implies. Again, we see this nascent movement to medicalize political issues, to overcome the American bias in favor of personal liberty and freedom of choice with epidemiological studies and grave men in white suits and the scolding finger of Big Brotherism. This is not what Hippocrates had in mind.

Nor did he quite envision C. Everett Koop. The man who came to Washington with such reluctance, the political naif who once saved handicapped infants and actually may have believed that to be a rewarding vocation, has long since metamorphosed into a (dare we say?) stout symbol of the corruption that seems to set in whenever a man stays too long in the corridors of political power.

But we may wonder if, as he races toward his ninth decade, Dr. Koop is at last content. The petty venalities and big payoffs of drkoop.com have perhaps sullied his reputation forever. He so sedulously built a reputation for incorruptible rectitude. After a few years in office, aided by a lapdog press, most of the country believed it. And now, after cashing in, he has everything he ever wanted—fame, riches, power—everything but reputation. His is shot. In the middle of the night, when a man's semi-conscious thoughts turn to his legacy, does Dr. C. Everett Koop regret what he has done? More importantly, will we?

Notes

Chapter 1

1. C. Everett Koop, *Koop: The Memoirs of America's Family Doctor* (New York: Random House, 1991), p. 149.
2. Margaret Carlson, "A Doctor Prescribes Hard Truth," *Time* (April 24, 1989), pp. 82–84.
3. Koop, *Koop*, p. 150.
4. Ibid., p. 316.
5. Ibid.
6. Mike McNamee and Geoffrey Smith, "Now It's C. Everett Koop Inc.: The Ex-Surgeon General is a Health-Education Conglomerate," *Business Week* (December 19, 1994), p. 36.
7. Koop, *Koop*, p. 27.
8. Ibid., p. 14.
9. Ibid., pp. 12–13.
10. Cory SerVaas, "The Surgeon General Is Determined: Interview with C. Everett Koop," *Saturday Evening Post* (April 1985), p. 52.
11. Koop, *Koop*, pp. 46–47.
12. Ibid., pp. 52–53.
13. Ibid., p. 62.
14. Ibid., p. 97.
15. Ibid., p. 87.
16. Ibid., p. 88.
17. Ibid., p. 127.
18. Ibid., p. 3.
19. Ibid., p. 5.
20. Ibid., p. 133.
21. Ibid., p. 140.
22. Fitzhugh Mullan, *Plagues and Politics: The Story of the United States Health Service* (New York: Basic Books, 1989), p. 134.
23. Ibid., p. 149.
24. Koop, *Koop*, p. 186.
25. Sheryl Gay Stolberg, "Job Itself in Doubt As New Feud Looms on Surgeon General," *New York Times*, February 5, 1998, p. A1.
26. Koop, *Koop*, p. 5.
27. Ibid., p. 6.

28. Ibid., p. 128.
29. Ibid., p. 148.
30. Ibid., p. 163.
31. Ibid., p. 167.
32. Ibid., p. 164.
33. Ibid., pp. 164–65.
34. Ibid., p. 191.
35. Ibid., pp. 173–74.
36. Ibid., p. 177.
37. Ibid.
38. Ibid., p. 180.
39. Ibid., p. 181.
40. Ibid., p. 184.
41. Quoted in Jacob Sullum, "Smoking and the Tyranny of Public Health," *Consumers' Research* (July 1998), p. 34.
42. Koop, *Koop*, p. 185.
43. Ibid., p. 167.
44. Ibid.
45. Jerry Berger, "'Unauthorized Biography' of Koop Is No Tell-All," *St. Louis Post-Dispatch*, October 13, 1991, p. 1C.
46. Carlson, "A Doctor Prescribes Hard Truth," pp. 82–84.
47. James Cox, "Koop's New Target: Alcohol," *USA Today*, May 31, 1989, p. 1B.
48. Koop, *Koop*, p. 298.
49. Randall Rothenberg, "Koop's Idea for Advertising Ban Debated," *New York Times*, February 14, 1990, p. D18.
50. G. Prince, "Koop Launches a Final Salvo on Alcohol with Drunk-Driving Report," *Beverage World* (June 30, 1989), p. 6.
51. Koop, *Koop*, p. 135.
52. Ibid., p. 314.
53. Gregg L. Cunningham, "Chicken Koop," *American Spectato*r (January 1994), p. 40.
54. Koop, *Koop*, p. 151.
55. Ibid., pp. 213–14.
56. Fran Pollner, "Dr. Koop Assesses His Record," *Medical World News* (July 10, 1989), p. 15.
57. Koop, *Koop*, pp. 215–16.
58. Ibid., pp. 222–23, 209.
59. Cunningham, "Chicken Koop," p. 41.
60. Koop, *Koop*, pp. 231–33.
61. Ibid., p. 312.
62. Ibid., p. 316.
63. Karen Pallarito, "Health Care Hall of Fame," *Modern Healthcare* (February 3, 1997), p. 38.
64. Koop, *Koop*, p. 316.
65. Rothenberg, *New York Times*, p. D18.
66. "Koop Continues to Speak Out," *The Alcoholism Report* (June 1992), p. 10.
67. Pallarito, *Modern Healthcare*, p. 38.
68. Daniel M. Gold, "Koop for the Defense," *Adweek's Marketing Week* (May 4, 1990), p. 6.
69. Robin Hoffman, "C. Everett Koop Stars in Biomedical Animal Research PSA," *Back Stage* (May 4, 1990), p. 26.

70. "Koop Leads," *Minneapolis Star-Tribune*, September 12, 1995, p. 3B.
71. Sabin Russell, "Health Plan Gets New Recruit—Koop," *San Francisco Chronicle*, September 21, 1993, p. A1.
72. "Breakfast at the White House: Koop Joins the Clintons and 100 Docs," *Health Line*, September 21, 1993.
73. "The Ethics of Health Care: An Interview with C. Everett Koop," *Christian Century* (January 26, 1994), p. 77.
74. "A Conversation with C. Everett Koop, M.D.," *Business & Health* (March 1992), p. 55.
75. Koop, *Koop*, pp. 34–36.
76. Russell, "Health Plan Gets New Recruit—Koop."
77. Craig D. Rose, "Koop Finds Flaws in Health Plan," *San Diego Union-Tribune*, May 5, 1994, p. C1.
78. "Koop Concerned About Managed Care," (Reuters), September 24, 1998, http:/ /www.pathfinder.com, p. 2.
79. "The Ethics of Health Care," *Christian Century*, p. 77.
80. Matt Kelley, "Hagel Criticizes Clinton on Burial Plot Waiver," *Omaha World-Herald*, February 3, 1998, p. 5.
81. Stephen Barr, "Panel Vows to Tighten Rules for Arlington Burial," *Washington Post*, January 29, 1998, p. A17.
82. "Hagel Criticizes Clinton on Burial Plot Waiver," *Omaha World-Herald*, p. 5.
83. Ibid.
84. "Koop Cedes Arlington Burial Claim," (Reuters) *Washington Post*, February 5, 1998.
85. Mike Yuen, "Koop: Use Settlement to Fight Tobacco," *Honolulu Star-Bulletin*, April 10, 1999.
86. "Koop Attacks GOP Congress As Being Pawns of Big Tobacco," *O'Dwyer's PR Services Report* (October 1998), p. 68.
87. Nancy Mathis, "Tobacco Remarks Burn Dole," *Houston Chronicle*, July 3, 1996, p. A1.
88. Mary McGrory, "The Unfitness Derby," *Washington Post*, July 7, 1996, p. C1.
89. "Koop: McCain Bill Soft on Tobacco," *National Journal's CongressDaily*, April 21, 1998.
90. "Morris: Tobacco Bill's Demise Yields Scant Dem Dividends," *National Journal's CongressDaily*, July 9, 1998.
91. Paul Bedard et al., "Wherefore Art Thou, Donor?" *U.S. News & World Report* (September 14, 1998), p. 7.
92. "Koop, Kessler Decline to Testify to Congress," *Washington Post*, March 5, 1998, p. A6.

Chapter 2

1. Jay Palmer, "Hey, Fatso!" *Barron's* (July 1, 1996), p. 25.
2. John Foreyt and Ken Goodrick, "The Ultimate Triumph of Obesity," *Lancet* (July 15, 1995), p. 134.
3. Berkeley Rice, "Can 'America's Family Doctor' Reshape Medical Education?" *Medical Economics* (January 25, 1993), p. 58.
4. John Tierney,"How to Get Rid of a Nag," *Hippocrates* (November 1988), p. 42.
5. Michael Fumento, *The Fat of the Land* (New York: Penguin, 1997), p. viii.
6. Palmer, *"Hey, Fatso!"*

7. Roberta Pollack Seid, *Never Too Thin: Why Women Are at War with Their Bodies* (New York: Prentice-Hall, 1989), pp. 3, 27.
8. Liz Brody, "The Diet Years," *Los Angeles Times*, February 1, 1996, p. E1.
9. Frances M. Berg, *Health Risks of Weight Loss*, 3rd. ed. (Hettinger, N.D.: *Healthy Weight Journal*, 1992), p. 14.
10. Quoted in ibid., p. 100.
11. Andrew Leckey, "Diet Industry Now Falling on Hard Times," *Baltimore Sun*, February 3, 1995, p. 9C.
12. "Pound Foolish," *People* (October 19, 1998), p. 119.
13. Jay Palmer, "Hey, Fatso!"
14. Lawrence Lindner, "Portion Distortion," *Washington Post Health*, November 3, 1998, p. 20.
15. William Bennett and Joel Gurin, *The Dieter's Dilemma*: *Eating Less and Weighing More* (New York: Basic Books, 1982), p. 172.
16. Ibid., p. 172.
17. Quoted in Hillel Schwartz, *Never Satisfied: A Cultural History of Diets, Fantasies and Fat* (New York: Free Press, 1986), p. 95.
18. Ibid., p. 95.
19. George F. Will, "Meg's Potent Measuredness," *Newsweek* (May 24, 1999), p. 83.
20. Schwartz, *Never Satisfied*, p. 96.
21. Fumento, *Fat of the Land*, p. 82.
22. Schwarz, *Never Satisfied*, pp. 142–143.
23. Seid, *Never Too Thin*, p. 99.
24. Ibid., p. 100.
25. Bennett and Gurin, *The Dieter's Dilemma*, p. 12.
26. Ibid., p. 14.
27. Ibid., p. 15.
28. Schwartz, *Never Satisfied*, p. 190.
29. Fumento, *Fat of the Land*, p. 3.
30. Fumento, *Fat of the Land*, p. 175.
31. Seid, *Never Too Thin*, p. 95.
32. Bennett and Gurin, *The Dieter's Dilemma*, p. 234.
33. Schwartz, *Never Satisfied*, p. 191.
34. Quoted in Fumento, *Fat of the Land*, p. 145.
35. Ibid., p. 143.
36. Seid, *Never Too Thin*, p. 168.
37. Schwartz, *Never Satisfied*, p. 309.
38. Bennett and Gurin, *The Dieter's Dilemma*, pp. 213–14.
39. Schwartz, *Never Satisfied*, p. 243.
40. James Langton, "Latest Way to Slim: Cut Off Your Stomach," *Daily Telegraph*, January 6, 1997, p. 23.
41. Fumento, *Fat of the Land*, p. 1.
42. Robinson G. Clark, "No More Fat City," *St. Louis Post-Dispatch*, January 30, 1994, p. 1E.
43. "Deception and Fraud in the Diet Industry, Part II," House of Representatives Committee on Small Business, May 7, 1990, Serial No. 101–57, p. 680.
44. Ibid., p. 680.
45. Berg, *Health Risks of Weight Loss*, pp. 101–102.
46. "Deception and Fraud in the Diet Industry, Part I," House of Representatives Committee on Small Business, March 26, 1990, Serial No. 101–50, p. 57.

47. Carol Krucoff, "Get Moving," *Washington Post*, August 12, 1997, p. Z10.
48. Berg, *Health Risks of Weight Loss*, p. 70.
49. Ibid., p. 73.
50. Ibid., p. 105.
51. Ibid., p. 18.
52. Ibid., p. 22.
53. Ibid., p. 139.
54. Ibid., p. 32.
55. Lawrence Lindner, "Eat, Drink and Be Healthy," *Washington Post Health*, February 2, 1999, p. 20.
56. Keith L. Alexander, "A Health Kick at Weight Watchers," *Business Week* (January 16, 1995), p. 36.
57. Stephen Baker, "Uh, Let's Think About That . . . " *Business Week* (September 22, 1997), p. 38.
58. Michael Lewis, "Royal Scam," *New York Times Magazine*, February 9, 1997, p. 22.
59. "Deception and Fraud in the Diet Industry, Part II," House of Representatives Committee on Small Business, May 7, 1990, Serial No. 101–57, p. 17.
60. Ibid., p. 18.
61. Ibid., p. 19.
62. Quoted in Fumento, *Fat of the Land*, p. 156.
63. Phyllis Berman and Amy Feldman, "Fat City," *Forbes* (February 17, 1992), p. 72.
64. Amy Barrett, "How Can Jenny Craig Keep Gaining?" *Business Week* (April 12, 1993), p. 52.
65. "Deception and Fraud in the Diet Industry, Part II," pp. 110–111.
66. Ibid., p. 590.
67. Ibid., p. 11.
68. "Deception and Fraud in the Diet Industry, Part I," p. 40.
69. "Deception and Fraud in the Diet Industry, Part II," p. 24.
70. "Juvenile Dieting, Unsafe Over-the-Counter Diet Products, and Recent Enforcement Efforts by the Federal Trade Commission," House of Representatives Committee on Small Business, September 24, 1990, Serial No. 101–80, p. 90.
71. Ibid., p. 218.
72. Clark, "No More Fat City."
73. Don Bauder, "Jenny Craig's Profits Drop As Does Client List," *San Diego Union-Tribune*, January 19, 1994, p. C1.
74. Margaret Carlson, "Public Eye," *Time* (December 12, 1994), p. 62.
75. "Weight Watchers in U.S. Agrees to Trim Bloated Success Stories," *Ottawa Citizen*, October 1, 1997, p. D4.
76. Cristina Rouvalis, "Weight Watchers Trims Work Force," *Pittsburgh Post-Gazette*, May 12, 1994, p. B10.
77. Chris Woodyard, "Heinz Plan Trims Weight Watchers," *USA Today*, March 17, 1997, p. 4B.
78. James Bernstein, "Weight Watchers Feels Corporate Belt-Tightening," *Newsday*, March 31, 1997, p. C3.
79. Barrett, "How Can Jenny Craig Keep Gaining?"
80. Fumento, *Fat of the Land*, p. 152.
81. "Deception and Fraud in the Diet Industry, Part IV" House of Representatives Committee on Small Business, May 21, 1992, Serial No. 102–78, p. 64.
82. Quoted in Berg, *Health Risks of Weight Loss*, p. 56.

83. Jenny Craig Inc., "Annual Report For the Fiscal Year Ended June 30, 1998," U.S. Securities and Exchange Commission, p. 9.
84. Fumento, *Fat of the Land*, p. 152.
85. Clark, "No More Fat City."
86. Seid, *Never Too Thin*, p. 280.
87. Ibid., pp. 280–81.
88. Laura Shapiro, "Is Fat That Bad?" *Newsweek* (April 21, 1997), pp. 58ff.
89. Carol Krucoff, "Get Moving."
90. Laura Shapiro, "Is Fat That Bad?"
91. Seid, *Never Too Thin*, p. 281.
92. Jay Palmer, "Hey, Fatso!"
93. Fumento, *Fat of the Land*, p. vii.
94. "Deception and Fraud in the Diet Industry, Part II," p. 679.
95. Ibid., pp. 682–83.
96. "Deception and Fraud in the Diet Industry, Part IV," p. 84.
97. "Deception and Fraud in the Diet Industry, Part I," p. 44.
98. "Deception and Fraud in the Diet Industry, Part IV," p. 120.
99. Jay Palmer, *Barron's*, p. 26.
100. "Deception and Fraud in the Diet Industry, Part IV," p. 106.
101. Quoted in Berg, *Health Risks of Weight Loss*, pp. 81–83.
102. Jerome P. Kassirer and Marcia Angell, "Losing Weight—An Ill-Fated New Year's Resolution," *New England Journal of Medicine* (January 1, 1998), p. 52.
103. Ibid., pp. 52–54.
104. Ibid., p. 53.
105. Quoted in Kathleen Fackelmann, "The Fat Fracas," *Science News* (May 2, 1998), p. 283.
106. Ibid.
107. Kassirer and Angell, "Losing Weight—An Ill-Fated New Year's Resolution."
108. Quoted in Jacob Sullum, "Smoking and the Tyranny of Public Health," *Consumers' Research* (July 1998), pp. 10ff.
109. Ibid.
110. "Arrest That Burger," *Washington Times*, September 15, 1995, editorial page.
111. Berg, *Health Risks of Weight Loss*, p. 36.
112. Fumento, *Fat of the Land*, p. 232.
113. Berg, *Health Risks of Weight Loss*, p. 36.
114. Fackelmann, "Fat Fracas."
115. "Deception and Fraud in the Diet Industry, Part II," p. 684.
116. Berg, *Health Risks of Weight Loss*, p. 105.
117. Bennett and Gurin, *The Dieter's Dilemma*, p. 211.
118. Seid, *Never Too Thin*, p. 12.
119. Krucoff, "Get Moving."
120. Fumento, *Fat of the Land*, p. 155.
121. Foreyt and Goodrick, "The Ultimate Triumph of Obesity."

Chapter 3

1. Jenny Craig Inc., "Annual Report to the Securities and Exchange Commission for the Fiscal Year Ending June 30, 1998," p. 8.
2. "What is Shape Up America?," http://www.shapeup.org, September 27, 1998, p. 1.

3. Abigail Trafford, "Winners and Losers: A Look at the Past Ten Years," *Washington Post*, January 3, 1995, p. Z1.
4. Laura Johannes and Steve Stecklow, "Dire Warnings about Obesity Rely on Slippery Statistic," *Wall Street Journal*, February 9, 1998, p. B1.
5. Ibid., p. B1.
6. Ibid.
7. Ibid., p. B8.
8. Brenda C. Coleman, "Study Fails to Confirm Fat, Breast Cancer Link," *Fairfax (Virginia) Journal*, March 10, 1999, p. A2.
9. Johannes and Stecklow, "Dire Warnings about Obesity," p. B8.
10. Nanci Hellmich, "Koop Kicks Off Shape-Up Program," *USA Today*, December 6, 1994, p. 1D.
11. Daniel Pinkwater, "President Clinton Needs a French Fry Fix," "All Things Considered," December 6, 1994.
12. Carol Wallace, "C. Everett Koop; After a Hostile Washington Welcome, a Contentious Surgeon General Has Become the Country's Most Visible and Aggressive Antismoking Crusader," *People* (April 21, 1986), pp. 91–95.
13. Ibid.
14. McNamee and Smith, *Business Week*, p. 36.
15. "Shape Up America," The Gale Group/Associations Unlimited, http://www.galenet.com, March 2, 1999.
16. "Shape Up America! Meet Dr. Koop and the Staff," http://www.shapeup.org, September 27, 1998.
17. "SUA Sponsors and How to Become One," http://www.shapeup.org, April 7, 1998.
18. "Wyeth's Redux, Mazanor Obesity Treatments Recommended for High to Extremely High Health Risk Patients," *Health News Daily* (October 31, 1996), p. 4.
19. Susan Milius, "FDA Approves New Fat Drug," UPI, April 29, 1996.
20. "What is Shape Up America?" http://www.shapeup.org, April 7, 1998.
21. "C. Everett Koop Declares War on Obesity," *The Bariatrician* (Fall 1996), cover.
22. "SUA 1996 Annual Report," http://www.shapeup.org, p. 18.
23. "Message from the Chairman," SUA 1996 Annual Report, http://www.shapeup.org, October 30, 1998.
24. "Program Structure," http://www.shapeup.org, April 7, 1998.
25. Steven Pratt, "Anti-Smoking Crusader Takes on Fat," *Chicago Tribune*, December 5, 1994, p. 1.
26. "Shaping Up," *Chicago Sun-Times*, January 1, 1995, p. 37.
27. "Jenny Craig Sponsors Dr. C. Everett Koop's 'Crusade' to Combat Obesity in America," PR Newswire, December 6, 1994.
28. Ibid.
29. Lee Martindale, "A Closer Look at 'Shape Up' Program," *Dallas Morning News*, November 15, 1996, p. 31A.
30. Shape Up America!/Special Advertising Feature, no date.
31. "Study Finds Weight Loss Can Be Maintained," Shape Up America!, October 1, 1997.
32. "Using Internet, Ex-Surgeon General Explains 'Cyberclinic' to Fight Obesity," *Chicago Tribune*, October 30, 1996, p. C7.
33. "SUA 1996 Annual Report," "Message from the Chairman."
34. Steven Pratt, "New Coup for Koop?" *Chicago Tribune*, December 15, 1994, p. C15.

35. Pratt, "Anti-Smoking Crusader Takes on Fat."
36. "Dr. C. Everett Koop Urges Business Community to Combat Obesity; Issues New Guide on Workplace Fitness," Shape Up America! press release, May 30, 1996.
37. *CNN Morning News,* October 30, 1996.
38. "Shape Up America! 1996 Annual Report," "TV Public Service Advertising Campaign" (not paginated).
39. "Informing Americans and Motivating Them to Act," ibid.
40. "Message from the Chairman," ibid.
41. "Dr. Koop Issues Action Plan to Implement the Surgeon General's Report on Physical Health and Activity," SUA Press release, July 11, 1996.
42. "Dr. C. Everett Koop Urges Congress to Tackle Causes of Preventable Deaths," PR Newswire, February 3, 1998.
43. "Dr. Koop Supports Goal to Increase Obesity Research," SUA press release, February 8, 1996.
44. Ibid.
45. "New Survey on Obesity and Body Image Finds That It's a Matter of Smoke and Mirrors," SUA press release, September 18, 1998.
46. "Anti-Diet Sentiment Is Pervasive," SUA press release, May 15, 1997.
47. Ira Dreyfuss, "Poor Lack Means to Exercise, Survey Says," *Los Angeles Times*, November 26, 1995, p. A28.
48. "Health Beat," *Plain Dealer* (Cleveland), May 28, 1996, p. 6E.
49. "Outdated Beliefs are Keeping Americans from Shaping Up," SUA press release, June 1, 1995.
50. "Low-Income Americans Face Major Obstacles to Weight Control, New Survey Finds," SUA press release, October 31, 1995.
51. "SUA 1996 Annual Report," "National Walking Campaign."
52. "Translating Goals into Action," http://www.shapeup.org.
53. "How Do You Measure BMI?" http://www.shapeup.org.
54. "Translating Goals into Action," "SUA 1996 Annual Report."
55. "The Costs of Obesity Are 'Staggering' But Women Are Paying the Highest Price, Says Dr. Koop," SUA press release, March 16, 1998.
56. Ibid.
57. Denise Mann, "Web Site Offers Hints on Dieting," *Arizona Republic*, May 29, 1997, p. HL4.
58. Ibid.
59. Ibid.
60. Jenny LaBalme, "Hoosiers Told of Obesity's Toll on Health," *Indianapolis Star*, June 6, 1998, p. B1.
61. "General Information," http://www.shapeup.org, April 7, 1998.
62. SUA 1996 Annual Report, "Message from the Chairman."
63. "AOA Mission Statement," Weight Wellness Week '98, Medeva Pharmaceuticals.
64. Statement of Judith S. Stern, American Obesity Association, House Subcommittee on Labor, Health and Human Resources, Education and Related Agencies, February 5, 1998.
65. "Welcome!" American Obesity Association, http://www.obesity.org, September 28, 1998.
66. Johannes and Stecklow, "Dire Warnings about Obesity." As bizarre as it may seem, this single member of the AOA may very well be Mattias Eng, our research assistant! When we gather information for our research on organiza-

tions such as the American Obesity Association, we arrange for our research assistants (or, in the case, of Shape Up America!, one of our wives under her maiden name) to join the group so that we routinely receive the mailings and other materials.

67. C. Everett Koop, "Obesity, An American Epidemic," *AOA Science Watch*, undated, p. 2.
68. Ibid., p. 1.
69. Dee J. Hall, "Fen-Phen Makers Fund Advocate," *Wisconsin State Journal*, April 5, 1998, p. 1A.
70. Ibid.
71. Morgan Downey, "Ground Zero in the Recall Wars," *AOA Report*, Vol. 1, No. 4, p. 2.
72. Hall, "Fen-Phen Makers Fund Advocate."
73. Ibid.
74. Nancy McVicar, "Fat Chance," Fort Lauderdale *Sun-Sentinel*, August 27, 1995, p. 1E.
75. Hall, "Fen-Phen Makers Fund Advocate."
76. "AOA Membership Application," undated.
77. "What is Obesity?" Weight Wellness Week brochure, revised August 25, 1998.
78. Hall, "Fen-Phen Makers Fund Advocate."
79. "FDA Introduces New Drug to Combat Obesity," *AOA Report*, Vol. 1, No. 4, p. 3.
80. "AOA Patient's Bill of Rights," *AOA Report*, Vol. 3, No. 1, p. 4.
81. "About the American Obesity Association," undated release.
82. "AOA Mission Statement," in "Welcome to Weight Wellness Week '98," p. 2.
83. "About the American Obesity Association."
84. "Wyeth's Redux, Mazanor Obesity Treatments Recommended for High to Extremely High Health Risk Patients."
85. "About the American Obesity Association."
86. "Weight Management and Health Insurance," American Obesity Association/ Knoll Pharmaceutical, 1998.
87. "Obesity Kills!" AOA press release, June 12, 1996.
88. See James T. Bennett and Thomas J. DiLorenzo, *The Food and Drink Police* (New Brunswick, N.J.: Transaction, 1999), pp. 93–100.
89. "AOA Seeks Greater Role for Obesity in Health Charter," *AOA Report*, Vol. 3, No. 1, pp. 1–3.
90. "Now There Is a Word for It," *AOA Report*, Vol. 1, No. 4, p. 7.
91. Downey, "Ground Zero in the Recall Wars," pp. 2, 8.
92. Steve Pratt, "Off Your Duff," *Chicago Tribune*, June 28, 1995, p. 3.
93. "Morgan Downey, CEO of the American Obesity Association," in Weight Wellness Week '98.
94. "A Note from the Executive Director," ibid.
95. Statement of Judith S. Stern, American Obesity Association, House Subcommittee on Labor, Health and Human Resources, Education and Related Agencies, February 5, 1998.
96. "Let's Give Obesity the Attention It Deserves," AOA, revised August 25, 1998.
97. "Childhood Obesity: A Growing Problem," *AOA Report*, Vol. 2, No. 1, p. 3.
98. "AOA Seeks Greater Role for Obesity in Health Charter," p. 4.
99. "Sticking With it: How to Avoid Becoming an Exercise Dropout," AOA, revised August 25, 1998.
100. "Price of Obesity Called Too High," (Knight-Ridder) Rochester, New York *Democrat & Chronicle*, September 16, 1999, p. 6A.

101. Mark D. Somerson, "Doctors Can't Ignore the Obese, Groups Say," *Columbus Dispatch* (Ohio), October 30, 1996, p. 3A.
102. "Guidance for Treatment of Adult Obesity," October 1996, http://shapeup.org.
103. Hall, "Fen-Phen Makers Fund Advocate."
104. Marion Nestle, "Alcohol Guidelines for Chronic Disease Prevention: From Prohibition to Moderation," *Nutrition Today* (March 13, 1997), pp. 86ff.
105. Lawrence Lindner, "Eat, Drink and Be Healthy," *Washington Post Health*, February 2, 1999, p. 20.
106. Sally Squires, "Optimal Weight Threshold Lowered," *Washington Post*, June 4, 1998, pp. A1–A13.
107. "Pound Foolish," *People* (October 19, 1998), p. 120.
108. Squires, "Optimal Weight Threshold Lowered."
109. "Development of the Weight Wellness Profile," *AOA Report*, Vol. 2, No. 2, p. 2.
110. Donna Britt, "Tipping the Scales Unkindly," *Washington Post*, June 5, 1998, p. B1.
111. Squires, "Optimal Weight Threshold Lowered."
112. Sally Squires, "Pound Foolish?" *Washington Post Health*, June 9, 1998, p. 6.
113. Laura Shapiro et al., "Is Fat That Bad?" *Newsweek* (April 21, 1997), p. 58.
114. "Obesity: Do the Math," ABCNEWS.com interact, undated.
115. Food and Drug Administration Drug Abuse, and Endocrinologic and Metabolic Drugs Advisory Committees Joint Meeting, Open Session, September 29, 1995, p. 46.
116. Richard Klein, "Leaning on Those Who Aren't Lean," *Wall Street Journal*, June 9, 1998, p. A18.
117. Stephen Goode, "Skinny on Fatty," *Insight* (December 2, 1996), p. 4.
118. "'Overweight' Category in New Guidelines Could Prompt Inappropriate Weight Loss—FDA Officials," *Blue Sheet* (June 24, 1998), p. 5.
119. Squires, "Optimal Weight Threshold Lowered."
120. Squires, "Pound Foolish?"
121. "Dr. Koop Calls on Overweight Americans to Become Patient Activists," SUA press release, September 4, 1997.
122. "First Obesity Treatment Guidelines Recommend All Treatment Options for High Health-Risk Patients," *Blue Sheet* (October 30, 1996).
123. F. Xavier Pi-Sunyer, "Obesity Research and Clinical Management," *Odyssey* (August 1998), http://www.glaxowellcome.com.

Chapter 4

1. Associated Press, September 28, 1995, untitled.
2. Laura Fraser, "The New Diet Drugs," *Health* (July 1996), p. 52.
3. Wendy Melillo, "Medication May Assist in Shedding Extra Pounds," *Washington Post*, March 9, 1993, p. Z13.
4. Gina Kolata, "How Fen-Phen, a Diet 'Miracle,' Rose and Fell," *New York Times*, September 23, 1997, p. F1.
5. McVicar, "Fat Chance."
6. Sally Squires, "Diet Pills Get a Second Look," *Washington Post*, December 6, 1994, p. Z14.
7. McVicar, "Fat Chance."

8. "Tracking the 'Fen-Phen' Drug Trend," *Physician and Sportsmedicine* (September 1996), p. 17.
9. Laura Fraser, "The New Diet Drugs."
10. Food and Drug Administration Endocrinologic and Metabolic Drugs Advisory Committee, Open Session, September 28, 1995, p. 47.
11. Wayne Biddle, "Profiting Off the Fat of the Land," *The Nation* (December 30, 1996), p. 20.
12. Nanci Hellmich, "New Appetite Regulator Approved," *USA Today*, April 30, 1996, p. 1A.
13. Food and Drug Administration Endocrinologic and Metabolic Drugs Advisory Committee, Open Session, November 16, 1995, p. 203.
14. Jay Palmer, *Barron's*, p. 28.
15. "Wyeth's Redux, Mazanor Obesity Treatments Recommended for High to Extremely High Health Risk Patients."
16. Food and Drug Administration Endocrinologic and Metabolic Drugs Advisory Committee, Open Session, September 28, 1995, p. 122.
17. David Kessler, "We've Fought the Good Fight," *Newsweek* (December 9, 1996), p. 28.
18. Food and Drug Administration Endocrinologic and Metabolic Drugs Advisory Committee, Open Session, September 28, 1995, p. 12.
19. Ibid.
20. Ibid., p. 14.
21. Ibid., pp. 15–16.
22. Ibid., pp. 16–19.
23. Ibid., p. 22.
24. Johannes and Stecklow, "Dire Warnings about Obesity."
25. Food and Drug Administration Endocrinologic and Metabolic Drugs Advisory Committee, Open Session, September 28, 1995, p. 24.
26. Ibid., p. 29.
27. Ibid., p. 38.
28. Ibid., pp. 40–41.
29. Ibid., pp. 55–56.
30. Ibid., p. 61.
31. Ibid., p. 88.
32. Ibid., pp. 79–80.
33. Ibid., p. 81.
34. Ibid., p. 102.
35. Ibid., p. 108.
36. Ibid., pp. 109–10.
37. Ibid., p. 151.
38. Ibid., p. 176.
39. Ibid., p. 140.
40. Ibid., pp. 242–43.
41. Ibid., p. 89.
42. Ibid., p. 126.
43. Ibid., p. 180.
44. Ibid., p. 182.
45. Fumento, *Fat of the Land*, p. 246.
46. Food and Drug Administration Endocrinologic and Metabolic Drugs Advisory Committee, Open Session, September 28, 1995, p. 190.

47. Ibid., p. 201.
48. Ibid., p. 204.
49. Ibid., p. 223.
50. Shari Roan, "Can These Pills Kill?" *American Health* (October 1996), p. 24.
51. Food and Drug Administration Endocrinologic and Metabolic Drugs Advisory Committee, Open Session, September 28, 1995, pp. 329–330.
52. Quoted in Food and Drug Administration Endocrinologic and Metabolic Drugs Advisory Committee, Open Session, November 16, 1995, p. 44.
53. Food and Drug Administration Endocrinologic and Metabolic Drugs Advisory Committee, Open Session, September 28, 1995, p. 180.
54. Kathleen Kerr, "Redux File Kept Secret," *Newsday*, February 16, 1998, p. A8.
55. Wayne Biddle, *Nation*, p. 20
56. Food and Drug Administration Endocrinologic and Metabolic Drugs Advisory Committee, Open Session, November 16, 1995, p. 11.
57. Ibid., p. 10.
58. Kerr, "Redux File Kept Secret."
59. Ibid., pp. 23–24.
60. Ibid., p. 61.
61. Ibid., p. 63.
62. Ibid., p. 84.
63. Ibid., p. 64.
64. Ibid., p. 248.
65. Ibid., p. 162.
66. Ibid., p. 170.
67. Ibid., p. 42.
68. Ibid., p. 43.
69. Ibid., p. 59.
70. Ibid., p. 30.
71. Ibid., pp. 244–45.
72. Ibid., pp. 252–53.
73. Hellmich, "New Appetite Regulator Approved."
74. Food and Drug Administration Drug Abuse, and Endocrinologic and Metabolic Drugs Advisory Committees Joint Meeting, Open Session, September 29, 1995, p. 15.
75. Ibid., p. 157.
76. *CNN Morning News*, January 3, 1997.
77. Roan, "Can These Pills Kill?"
78. Dana Canedy, "Weight Loss from Out of a Bottle," *New York Times*, February 14, 1997, p. D1.
79. Food and Drug Administration Drug Abuse, and Endocrinologic and Metabolic Drugs Advisory Committees Joint Meeting, Open Session, September 29, 1995, p. 21.
80. "Jenny Craig Annual Report to the SEC for Fiscal Year Ending June 30, 1998," p. 4.
81. Canedy, "Weight Loss from Out of a Bottle."
82. Kolata, "How Fen-Phen, a Diet 'Miracle,' Rose and Fell."
83. Morgan Downey, "Ground Zero in the Recall Wars," p. 2.
84. McVicar, "Fat Chance."
85. Greg Johnson, "Scales Tip Toward Drug-Free Weight Loss," *Los Angeles Times*, September 17, 1997, p. D3.
86. Hellmich, "New Appetite Regulator Approved."

87. Canedy, "Weight Loss from Out of a Bottle."
88. Laura Johannes and Steve Stecklow, "Sales of Diet Pills Plunge As Health Concerns Are Raised," *San Diego Union-Tribune*, September 8, 1997, p. C3.
89. John Schwartz, "2 Diet Drugs are Pulled Off Market," *Washington Post*, September 16, 1997, p. A1.
90. Kitta MacPherson and Edward R. Silverman, "Diet Pill Saga," *Chicago Tribune*, October 12, 1997, p. 8, *Womanews*.
91. Brooke A. Masters, "Va. Woman Settles with Diet Drug Firm," *Washington Post*, December 8, 1998, p. D3.
92. Johannes and Stecklow, "Sales of Diet Pills Plunge."
93. Ed Hayward, "Diet to Death," *Boston Herald*, May 6, 1997, p. 1.
94. Kathleen Kerr, "Fen-Phen & Deaths," *Newsday*, October 19, 1997, p. A5.
95. "What Has AOA Done?" Weight Wellness Week '98.
96. Food and Drug Administration Drug Abuse, and Endocrinologic and Metabolic Drugs Advisory Committees Joint Meeting, Open Session, September 29, 1995, p. 18.
97. Kathleen Doheny, "Getting to the Heart of the Matter After Recall of Drugs," *Los Angeles Times*, September 22, 1997, p. S6.
98. Whitney Walker and Sallie Han, "The Pills and the Pendulum," *Daily News*, November 2, 1997, p. 44.
99. Morgan Downey, "Ground Zero in the Recall Wars," p. 1.
100. "In Spite of Diet Drug Withdrawal, The War on Obesity Must Continue, Says Dr. Koop," SUA press release, September 19, 1997.
101. Sandra G. Boodman, "Just One New Diet Drug on the Horizon," *Washington Post Health*, January 5, 1999, p. 9.
102. Anna Mulrine, "The Scramble to Develop a Miracle Diet Drug," *U.S. News & World Report* (February 15, 1999), p. 44.
103. Sandra G. Boodman, "Just One New Diet Drug on the Horizon."

Chapter 5

1. Mike McNamee and Geoffrey Smith, "Now, It's C. Everett Koop, Inc.," *Business Week* (December 19, 1994), p. 36.
2. "C. Everett Koop, Former Surgeon General, Joins Mbf USA, Inc. as Chairman of the Board," *Business Wire*, May 17, 1994.
3. Ibid.
4. "Mbf USA Inc. Reports Highest Quarterly Profits in Its History," *Business Wire*, July 25, 1994.
5. Russell Shaw, "Egg Campaign to Roll Out," *Supermarket News*, (February 5, 1996), p. 17.
6. Robert Pool, "Slow Going for Blood Substitutes," *Science* (December 21, 1990), p. 4988.
7. BioPure press release, December 2, 1997.
8. Pool, "Slow Going for Blood Substitutes."
9. "Philanthropy Notes," *Foundation Watch* (Washington, D.C.: Capital Research Center, August 1999), p. 10.
10. John Maggs, "Money Greases Massive Effort to Protect Glaxo Windfall," *Journal of Commerce*, October 25, 1995, p. 3A.
11. John Maggs, "Koop Says He Was Unaware of Details of Glaxo Ad," *Journal of Commerce*, December 4, 1995, p. 1A.

12. "Glaxo Defends Lobbying Effort," *Journal of Commerce*, October 30, 1995, p. 1A.
13. "C. Everett Koop: Calls on Patients to Empower Themselves," *Health Line*, September 16, 1996.
14. Holcomb B. Noble, "Koop Criticized for Role in Warning on Hospital Gloves," *New York Times*, October 29, 1999.
15. "The Tarnished Image of Dr. Koop," *Chicago Tribune*, October 30, 1999.
16. "Koop to Help First Circle Develop Hyperthermia System," *Medical Industry Today*, January 13, 1998.
17. "First Circle Medical Personnel: Management Profile," http://www.fcmedical. com.
18. Dick Youngblood, "First Circle Tries to Advance 'Fever Therapy' Technology," Minneapolis *Star Tribune*, April 13, 1998, p. 2D.
19. *Medical Industry Today*, January 13, 1998.
20. Ibid.
21. Youngblood, "First Circle Tries to Advance 'Fever Therapy' Technology."
22. Ronald H. Lane, "To Our Shareholders," *1998 Bionutrics Annual Report*.
23. "Bionutrics Annual Report to the Securities and Exchange Commission for the Fiscal Year Ending October 31, 1997," p. 7.
24. "Notice of Annual Meeting of Stockholders for the Year Ended October 31, 1998 to be Held on March 30, 1999," Bionutrics, Inc., p. 8.
25. "Bionutrics Annual Report to the Securities and Exchange Commission for the Fiscal Year Ended October 31, 1998," p. 19.
26. "Neurocrine Biosciences, Inc., Annual Report to the Securities and Exchange Commission for the Fiscal Year Ended December 31, 1997," p. 8.
27. David F. Saks, Adam Greene, and David Weiner, "Neuocrine Biosciences, Inc.," Gruntal Investment Research, September 29, 1997.
28. "Time Life Inc. and C. Everett Koop Join Forces to Create First Comprehensive, Mass-Marketed Patient Education Videos," Business Wire, November 28, 1994.
29. Ellen Joan Pollock, "Tales of the Tapes: How One Media Deal Became Hazardous to Investors' Health," *Wall Street Journal*, February 13, 1997, p. A1.
30. "Welcome to the Koop Foundation Home Page," Koop Foundation, Inc., http://www.koopfoundation.org.
31. Ibid.
32. Sabin Russell, "Health Plan Gets New Recruit," *San Francisco Chronicle*, September 21, 1993, p. A1.
33. "Welcome to the Koop Foundation Home Page," http://www.koopfoundation.org.
34. Ibid.
35. Ibid.
36. "Target Outcomes," Koop Foundation, Inc. HII Project IRB/TRB, Koop Award ATP-1 Releasable Documents.
37. "Welcome to the Koop Foundation Home Page," http://www.koopfoundation.org.
38. "HOLON Pilot Site Case Studies," High Performance Healthcare . . . An Advanced Technology Program Review of HOLON, Koop Award 5H1191 ATP-2 Releaseable Documents.
39. "About the ATP," NIST Home Page, http://www.atp.nist.gov.
40. "Important Facts," NIST Home Page, http://www.atp.nist.gov.
41. "About the ATP," http://www.atp.nist.gov.
42. "Healthcare System Performance Issues," Koop Foundation, Inc. HII Project IRB, TRB, Koop Award ATP-1 Releasable Documents.

43. "About the ATP," http://www.atp.nist.gov.
44. "Consumers and Health Informatics," House of Representatives Subcommittee on Human Resources and Intergovernmental Relations, July 26, 1996, p. 41.
45. Ibid., p. 6.
46. Ibid., p. 10.
47. "About the ATP," http://www.atp.nist.gov.
48. "Clarification to Form CD-511," Koop Award 5H1012 Folder 1.
49. e-mail from carlson@sst.ncsl.nist.gov to Donna Jean Garrett, March 17, 1995, Koop Award 5H1012 Folder 2.
50. Donna Jean Garrett to NBSMICF (BJLIDE), March 10, 1995, Koop Award 5H1012 Folder 2.
51. Donna Jean Garrett to NBSMICF (BJLIDE), February 23, 1995, Koop Award 5H1012 Brown Folder 8.
52. E-mail from Teresa Farris to Mdmkfi@aol.com, March 26, 1997, Koop Award 5H1012 Folder 1.
53. E-mail from Teresa Farris to barbara.lambis@nist.gov, April 3, 1997, Koop Award 5H1012 Folder 2.
54. E-mail from Gwen Simpson to Teresa Farris, April 7, 1997, Koop Award 5H1012 Folder 2.
55. E-mail from jwow@micf.nist.gov to Michelle A. Sullivan, May 23, 1996, Koop Award ATP-4.
56. Note from Donna Jean Garrett to NBSMICF (BJLIDE), February 7, 1995, Koop Award 5H1012 Folder 2.
57. Memo from Teresa Farris, February 25, 1998, Koop Award 5H1012 Folder 3.
58. Note from Brian Belanger to Donna Jean Garrett, January 19, 1995, Koop Award 5H1012 Folder 2.
59. E-mail from Donna Jean Garrett to brianb@enh.nist.gov, January 19, 1995, ibid.
60. E-mail from Teresa Farris to leedy@micf.nist.gov, April 1, 1997, Koop Award ATP-1.
61. Letter from Koop Foundation Inc. (author blacked out) to Bettijoyce B. Lide, NIST, April 29, 1997, Koop Award 5H1191 Folder 2.
62. Handwritten note by Teresa Farris, August 1, 1998, Koop Award 5H1191 Folder 4.
63. E-mail to bettijoyce.lide@nist.gov (sender blacked out), April 24, 1997, Koop Award 5H1191 ATP-2.
64. E-mail from bettyijoyce.lide@nist.gov (recipient blacked out), April 25, 1997, ibid.
65. E-mail from Doug Foellmer@koopfoundation.org to numerous recipients, August 5, 1998, Koop Award ATP-3.
66. "Summary—C. Everett Koop Institute 94–04–0037," no author given, January 25, 1999, ibid.
67. Holcomb B. Noble, "Scientist at Work: C. Everett Koop; He's 'Gone Commercial' to Spread Gospel of Health," *New York Times*, February 2, 1999.
68. Berkeley Rice, "Can 'America's Family Doctor' Reshape Medical Education?" *Medical Economics* (January 25, 1993), p. 58.
69. "The C. Everett Koop Institute," http://koop.dartmouth.edu., October 16, 1998.
70. "Hepatitis C: An Epidemic for Anyone," ibid., October 23, 1998.
71. "Hepatitis C Awareness," ibid.
72. Noble, "Scientist at Work: C. Everett Koop."

73. "Dr. Francis J. Tedesco, President of the Medical College of Georgia, Elected to the Board of A.D.A.M. Software, Inc.," PR Newswire, July 25, 1996.
74. "Item 3. Legal Proceedings," http://www.sec.gov/Archives/edgar/data, March 24, 1999, p. 1.
75. Charles Piller, "Intel Sees Internet Health Initiative As a Tonic to PC Sales," *Los Angeles Times*, October 26, 1998, p. C4.
76. "Intel: Launches Ambitious Internet Health Initiative," *Health Line*, October 29, 1998.
77. Charles Piller, "Intel Sees Internet Health Initiative As a Tonic to PC Sales."
78. "Intel: Launches Ambitious Internet Health Initiative."
79. "Superior Consultant Holdings Introduces Consumer Health Initiative With Empower Health Corporation," PR Newswire, May 4, 1998.
80. "About Empower Health," http://www.empowerhealth.com, November 5, 1998.
81. "Superior Consultant Holdings Corporation Welcomes Former U.S. Surgeon General Dr. C. Everett Koop to Its Board of Directors," PR Newswire, May 28, 1998.
82. "Superior Consultant Holdings Introduces Consumer Health Initiative With Empower Health Corporation."
83. "Richard Helppie, Chairman of Superior Consultant Holdings Corporation, Joins Empower Health Board," Business Wire, May 28, 1998.
84. "Superior Consultant Holdings Corporation Welcomes Former U.S. Surgeon General Dr. C. Everett Koop to Its Board of Directors."
85. "Superior Banking on Koop Name with Investment," *Health Data Network News*, May 20, 1998.
86. Superior Consultant Holdings Corporation, Schedule 14A: Information Required in Proxy Statement, p. 16.
87. "Corporate Profile: Superior Consultant Holdings Corporation," http://www.superiorconsultant.com, November 5, 1998.
88. Richard D. Helppie, ibid.
89. "Dr. C. Everett Koop Announces Prevention Initiative on the Web," PR Newswire, November 5, 1998.
90. Stacey Schultz, "No Miracle Cure," *U.S. News & World Report* (August 10, 1998), p. 65.
91. Ibid.
92. "Using Thermometers," Dr. Koop's Community, http://www.drkoop.com, November 5, 1998.
93. "US Waistlines: Super Sized," Reuters, May 28, 1998.
94. "drkoop.com and Health Resources Publishing Company Maximize the Patient/Pharmacist Relationship," PR Newswire, March 10, 1999.
95. "About Empower Health," http://www.empowerhealth.com, November 5, 1998.
96. "Privacy Policy," http://www.drkoop.com, October 23, 1998.
97. "Sponsorship: Advertising and Sponsorship Opportunities," http://www.empowerhealth.com, November 5, 1998.
98. Search for "Smoking," http://www.drkoop.com, November 5, 1998.
99. "Dr. Koop's Community Partner Program Provides Trusted Online Patient Education and Interactive Capabilities to Healthcare Organizations," PR Newswire, October 26, 1998.
100. Matt Labash, "Dr. Koop Sells Himself," *Weekly Standard* (July 5/12, 1999), p. 29.
101. "New Site Redesign Supports Brand Strategy," PR Newswire, March 29, 1999.
102. Labash, "Dr. Koop Sells Himself."

103. Ibid., p. 29.
104. John Schwartz, "Just Call Him Doc.Com: Koop's Web IPO Clicks," *Washington Post*, June 9, 1999, p. A10.
105. Labash, "Dr. Koop Sells Himself."
106. "Koop: Making $$$ From Web Site," The Hotline (*National Journal*), March 9, 1999.
107. Mark Leibovich, "Here.com the Celebrities," *Washington Post*, June 10, 1999, p. E1.
108. "Overall Technical Goals and Interim Milestones," KFI-ATP1 Project Continuation and Carryover of Funds for Year 3, Koop Award ATP 1.
109. Ann Carrns, "Reflecting Trust in Ex-Surgeon General, Drkoop.com Raises $84.4 Million in IPO," *Wall Street Journal*, June 9, 1999, p. B8.
110. Alan Abelson, "Oh, Doctor!" *Barron's*, June 14, 1999, p. 3.
111. John Schwartz, "Auditors Question drkoop.com's Health," *Washington Post*, April 1, 2000; John Schwartz, "5 Months Left for drkoop.com," *Washington Post*, April 26, 2000.
112. Holcomb B. Noble, "Hailed as Surgeon General, Koop Criticized on Web Ethics," *New York Times*, September 5, 1999, pp. A1, A18.
113. "Special Note from Dr. Koop," http://www.drkoop.com, September 6, 1999.
114. Labash, "Dr. Koop Sells Himself."

Chapter 6

1. "Obesity Is Soaring in America," Associated Press, October 26, 1999.
2. Bennett and DiLorenzo, *The Food and Drink Police*.
3. Cori Vanchieri, "Lessons from the Tobacco Wars Edify Nutrition War Tactics," *Journal of the National Cancer Institute* (March 18, 1998), pp. 420–22.
4. Ibid.

Index